After Miscarriage

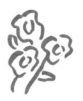

After Miscarriage

MEDICAL FACTS AND EMOTIONAL SUPPORT FOR PREGNANCY LOSS

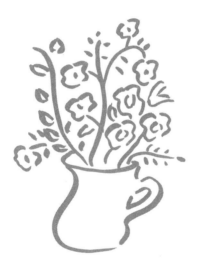

KRISSI DANIELSSON

FOREWORD BY WILLIAM H. KUTTEH, M.D., PH.D., H.C.L.D.

The Harvard Common Press

Boston, Massachusetts

The Harvard Common Press
535 Albany Street
Boston, Massachusetts 02118
www.harvardcommonpress.com

Printed in the United States of America
Printed on acid-free paper

Library of Congress Cataloging-in-Publication Data

Danielsson, Krissi.
   After miscarriage : medical facts and emotional support for pregnancy
loss / Krissi Danielsson.
       p. cm.
   Includes bibliographical references and index.
   ISBN-13: 978-1-55832-353-7 (hardcover : alk. paper)
   ISBN-13: 978-1-55832-354-4 (pbk. : alk. paper)
   1. Miscarriage—Popular works.   I. Title.
   RG648.D32 2008
   618.3'92—dc22

                                                      2007025893

Special bulk-order discounts are available on this and other Harvard
Common Press books. Companies and organizations may purchase
books for premiums or resale, or may arrange a custom edition,
by contacting the Marketing Director at the address above.

Book design by Jill Weber
Cover illustration by Lane duPont

10 9 8 7 6 5 4 3 2 1

For MATT

I told you I was going to dedicate this to someone else,

but this book wouldn't be here without you.

I love you.

And don't say, "You'd better, dammit."

Contents

If You're Buying This Book for a Friend or Loved One . . .

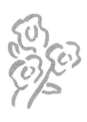

IF YOU'VE NEVER BEEN THROUGH A MISCARRIAGE yourself, or even if you have, it can be hard to know what to say to someone who has just had one. As part of the research for this book, I asked women to discuss what people did for them that helped the most, and what others said that unintentionally hurt. Here are some of the comments:

WHAT HELPED:

Most people listened and told me that they knew others who had miscarried, and one friend revealed she had had a miscarriage, too, so I felt I was not alone.

—MARY

Friends who had gone through similar experiences called me to talk or offered a shoulder to cry on. My bishop also made time for me.

—RHONDA

A friend has given me all her baby gear. Her belief that I will again have a pregnancy, and that it will result in a healthy baby, helps.

—TINA

A few people sent cards, and to this day my mother sends me cards on Mother's Day. It helped to have the losses acknowledged.

— ANITA

Just being there to let me talk, and not judging how I felt, was the best thing people did for me. One friend bought a beautiful house-plant for us; we really appreciated that.

—DESIREE

My boss gave me two weeks off and paid me for them; I didn't have to use sick leave or vacation time.

—SHERRY

I received many phone calls from people in our church. It helped to know people were thinking of me and praying for me.

—CASSANDRA

My best friend came over, and we sat and talked about everything. My hopes and dreams for that child were all spoken that day, and we even named the baby. We laughed and we cried together; she shared all my emotions.

—TAMMY

One friend brought dinner to my house and arranged for dinner to be sent over by others for three more nights.

—GISELLE

Another couple came to the hospital after my D&C with my favorite chocolate dessert! During my second loss, my doctor called me every day for a week and offered me his ear. That helped a lot.

—HANNAH

WHAT NOT TO SAY:

Many couples who experience miscarriages are subjected to thoughtless comments from people who probably mean well but don't understand that what they're saying not only doesn't help but may hurt the feelings of someone who has miscarried. Here are some examples of things you should not say to someone who has had a miscarriage:

- It was for the best.

- At least you know you can get pregnant.

- Something was probably wrong with it.

- Maybe God knows you're not ready to have children.

- You're trying too hard. Just relax, and it will happen.

- Take my kids for an afternoon, and I promise you won't be so sad about losing the baby.

- Maybe you should get a dog instead; they're so much easier to take care of.

- Be glad. Having a baby changes your life; think of all the fun things you wouldn't have been able to do anymore.

- You should just be happy you have one/two/three children already. You don't need any more.

- It was just a blob of cells. It wasn't a real baby.

- You're young. You'll get pregnant again.

- It happens all the time; it's nothing to worry about.

- At least you weren't very far along.

- It just wasn't meant to be.

- It probably happened because _____.

Preface

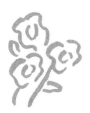As you probably have noticed, medical practitioners and psychologists write most of the health-oriented books on the market. So one of the first things that may strike you when you pick up this book is that I am not a physician. I'm not a psychologist, either, although I do have an undergraduate degree in the field. At the time of this writing, I do not hold any kind of medical credential.

My perspective on miscarriage is that of a mother. I had three miscarriages in a period of 14 months when my husband and I started trying to build our family. These were my first experiences with a medical system that I had previously believed was infallible and held the answers to all health ills. When you're not a regular user of the health care system, it's easy to think that there are no more medical frontiers, that modern medicine understands the human body fairly well. I soon learned this is not the case. Although much progress has been made, many medical mysteries remain. One of these is recurrent miscarriage.

After my losses I embarked on a research mission, the first of many for me. This book is what I wish had been available when I first started on this journey—a simple, unbiased collection of the known facts about miscarriage causes and treatments, followed by a discussion of coping strategies you can use as you proceed with your life. Writing this book brought back many painful memories, but I hope that it will help a lot of people.

This book should not serve as a substitute for a physician's advice. Medical decisions are individual, and yours should be made with your practitioner. Rather than being prescriptive, this book is meant to inform and empower you—to give you ideas to explore with your practitioner and to help you proceed more confidently with your attempts to build your family.

I know this book can't be all things to all people. Because I experienced multiple miscarriages, I am especially sensitive to the needs of others who have had more than one pregnancy loss. If you are picking up this book after your first miscarriage, please do not be alarmed by the discussion of miscarriage causes, and please keep in mind that, after a single miscarriage, the odds are very high that the next pregnancy will be successful.

For those who have suffered multiple losses, this book will provide information about possible causes and tests that you can ask about, as well as potential treatments and current research that may result in new treatments for recurrent miscarriage.

For readers who have experienced one or several miscarriages, I also discuss the emotional aspects of coping and facing the world while grieving. When you are ready to try again, I hope you will benefit from the tips here for handling the anxiety you may experience both before and after you conceive.

Throughout the book I have included comments by women who have had pregnancy losses, and who share their feelings and offer suggestions for how to get through this painful time. I hope that these comments will let you know that you are not alone and that what you are feeling is normal. If you visit the Web site for this book, www.aftermiscarriage.com, you will find a selection of stories by women who had miscarriages and then successfully carried pregnancies to term. I hope these stories will inspire you and remind you that your story, too, will most likely have a happy ending someday.

The medical research for this book was conducted through interviews with medical practitioners and by using online databases of medical journal articles. I've cited sources throughout, and I have had the medical information in this book reviewed by a physician for technical accuracy.

During my journey through recurrent miscarriage and some personal experiences that followed, I have become a believer in some forms of alternative medicine, so I am including information about alternative treatments for miscarriage that you can use as you see fit. In managing your health, you alone are in the driver's seat.

Whatever your individual circumstances, may this book bring you comfort and help you along throughout your own journey. Please feel free to e-mail me at author@aftermiscarriage.com with your comments.

Acknowledgments

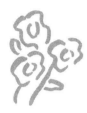 My thanks go out to the following health professionals and researchers for their interview comments that are included in this book:

- Mark P. Leondires, M.D., F.A.C.O.G., medical director and lead physician, Reproductive Medicine Associates of Connecticut

- Paolo Rinaudo, M.D., Ph.D., assistant professor of reproductive endocrinology and infertility, University of California, San Francisco

- Barry Jacobs, M.D., F.A.C.O.G., Texas Fertility, P.A.

- Kristen Swanson, R.N., Ph.D., F.A.A.N., professor and chair, Department of Family and Child Nursing, University of Washington

- Denise Côté-Arsenault, Ph.D., R.N.C., University of Rochester School of Nursing.

- Melinda Olson, R.N., B.S.N., cofounder, president, and Mama in Charge, Earth Mama Angel Baby herbal-products company

- Gerald Williams, L.Ac. (California), D.A. (Rhode Island), M.S.T.O.M., clinical director and founder, Reproductive Wellness

- Madeline Licker Feingold, Ph.D., clinical psychologist specializing in reproductive medicine, Berkeley, California

And an extra huge thank-you to Patricia Robertson, M.D., professor of clinical obstetrics and gynecology and specialist in maternal-fetal medicine at the University of California, San Francisco, and William H.

Kutteh, M.D., Ph.D., H.C.L.D., director of Fertility Associates of Memphis, Memphis Fertility Laboratory, and Reproductive Laboratory, for giving the book a medical reality check.

Thanks also to all the readers of the BellaOnline miscarriage Web site, who helped by filling out my miscarriage survey form and sharing their innermost feelings about this heartbreaking experience.

Thanks to the women who shared their stories about overcoming miscarriage and to the three poets who agreed to let me publish their work in this book to help other women get through this experience.

Thanks to Jacky Sach for her help and advice.

Thanks to Linda Ziedrich for her insightful comments and suggestions during the editing process.

Thanks also to my husband, Matt, and to my parents, Jeff and Lori Pulliam, for the unconditional support that they have always given me.

Foreword

By William H. Kutteh, M.D., Ph.D., H.C.L.D.

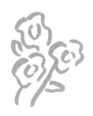 Krissi Danielsson suffered one of the most profound personal tragedies that people seeking parenthood face: recurrent pregnancy loss. In *After Miscarriage*, Danielsson has created a resource that should be useful to any couple dealing with the repercussions of miscarriage. She has carefully recorded and analyzed her experiences, and has added comments from other women who have dealt with the unexpected heartache of pregnancy loss. The author has also performed considerable research, both with patients and health-care providers; her up-to-date summary of medical facts provides excellent information to couples.

Spontaneous abortion occurs in approximately 15 to 20 percent of clinically diagnosed pregnancies of reproductive-aged women, and recurrent pregnancy loss occurs in about 3 to 5 percent of this same population. A definite cause of recurrent pregnancy loss can be established in approximately two-thirds of couples after a thorough evaluation. Krissi Danielsson helps readers determine when they need a specialist and when to seek additional testing, and she deals with the difficult issue of insurance coverage for some of the expensive tests that may be recommended. (A complete evaluation will include investigations into genetic, hormonal, anatomic, immunologic, infectious, thrombophilic, and environmental causes.) Couples faced with pregnancy loss may also encounter significant emotional distress, and in some cases supportive care may be necessary; Danielsson shares some of the strategies that have worked for her and other couples.

The book's eight chapters begin with acknowledgment of a woman's feelings when her baby is gone and move into discussions of the known causes of recurrent pregnancy loss. Danielsson includes information on medical testing and treatments as well as alternative therapies that help with stress reduction. Next she takes the reader through the experience of coping with pregnancy loss and building up the strength to try again. Her husband, Matt, adds his thoughts as well as those of other men who are dealing with the loss of the pregnancy and the grief in their relationship. Finally, there is a very useful glossary of medical terms commonly encountered in discussions of miscarriage and a list of helpful online resources.

I recommend *After Miscarriage* for couples who have experienced recurrent pregnancy loss and need answers. The book will empower such couples to seek information and testing to uncover the possible cause of their losses and help them gain the strength to try again.

After Miscarriage

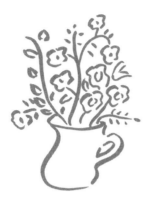

THE MISCARRIAGE

by Linda Wasmer Andrews

There has been a death in the family.
There has been a death in the family.

No eulogy, no coffin,
No funeral, no black.

And yet, there has been a death in the family.

No undertaker, no hearse,
No cemetery, no grave.

And yet, there has most assuredly been a
death in the family.

No belly, no fullness
No lifeline, no baby.

There has been a death in the family.

CHAPTER 1

My Baby Is Gone

I OFFER YOU MY CONDOLENCES for having felt compelled to pick up this book. You are probably feeling alone and in a place that no one should ever have to be.

A lot of articles about miscarriage start with some variation of a bone-headed statement like "Miscarriage can be the most devastating experience in a woman's life." Pick up a miscarriage support book, and you'll likely find yourself reading an anecdote about an average couple who were devastated to learn of a pregnancy loss, followed by the author's trite explanation that miscarriages are common and usually nothing to worry about.

I've always hated that.

This book is different. You already know how devastated you were to learn of your miscarriage, and no one needs to tell you that it's a terrible thing to experience. You've probably already heard the speech about how miscarriages are as common as the common cold and how one miscarriage rarely means anything is wrong with a woman. But you may not have found this speech entirely reassuring. If you were lucky, your practitioner may have taken the time to explain everything to you in a sensitive manner that left you feeling truly hopeful about your chances for conceiving children in the future. If not, you may find yourself feeling alone in the quest for answers amid a sea of questions and confusion. If this was your first miscarriage, or if you've had more than one but are still unsure what happened, I hope this chapter will be a starting point to help you understand and sort everything out.

How I Came to Write This Book

My own experience with miscarriages spanned an almost two-year period from April 2001 until my daughter's birth in February 2003. The experience turned my life upside down and continues to shape the person I am today.

I suffered my first miscarriage in July 2001. Although we had thrown out the birth control pills two months before, my husband and I had just barely processed the fact that I was pregnant. Pregnancy seemed like an abstract concept until that second line appeared on the home pregnancy test. I went to a walk-in clinic to confirm the pregnancy. But something was wrong.

The first sign there was a problem came when the nurse told me the urine pregnancy test was negative. We stared at her, dumbfounded, while she went to check it again. Why would it have been negative when the test at home had been so clearly positive just hours earlier? She returned to say the result was now a faint positive. The clinic's doctor ordered a blood test to check the level of pregnancy hormone. That afternoon, he called to say that the level was 50 and that I should come back in two days for a follow-up blood test. Something in the doctor's tone gave me the distinct feeling that it wasn't time to celebrate.

After the second blood test, which showed a level of 63, the clinic's obstetrician-gynecologist called and told me that I was "probably going to miscarry" and that I should expect a "crampy" period, but that this was nothing to worry about. She didn't seem to think anything was amiss with me, and she left me with hope that the pregnancy could still turn out okay. The uncertainty of my situation only made it harder.

I spent the next several days in shock, bursting into tears throughout the day for no apparent reason. I checked my underwear for spots of blood about 20 times a day. My husband kept telling me not to worry, that things would turn out fine.

Several months before, we had booked a vacation for that week, so we tried to leave our concerns at home as we headed to the airport. When we'd learned I was pregnant, the vacation had seemed like a beautiful way to celebrate the life transition that was coming—a nice week with just the two of us and the new life growing inside me. I tried my best to maintain my composure and not think the worst. My husband even patted my belly when the flight attendant announced an early-boarding call for passengers with small children. But the bleeding started by the time we reached our destination.

The vacation went downhill from there.

When we returned home a week later with the bleeding nearly complete, I wasn't sure what to do. I probably should have called the doctor I'd seen before, but instead I went to the walk-in clinic and told the on-call doctor what had happened. He rolled his eyes and insisted it was normal, and then offered to prescribe mood-altering drugs if I was unable to handle my emotions. Everything would be fine next time, he said; miscarriage was just a part of life and nothing to worry about.

For most women, after one miscarriage the next pregnancy really is fine. But in my case, the next pregnancy wasn't fine; nor was the one after that. The doctor was right, though, that miscarriage was a part of life, for me, from that point on.

The next time I got pregnant, bleeding started at nine weeks, and an ultrasound test showed that the baby had stopped growing at six weeks, so I opted for a D&C (dilation and curettage; see pages 8 and 13) to speed the process. The week between when the bleeding started and the D&C was completed was probably the worst in my life. No one could tell me for sure whether my baby had died, and the medical staff insisted on maintaining a rosy outlook even when the evidence was clear. The ultrasound technician even insisted my dates were wrong, although the pregnancy had been confirmed early on.

I went on to have another loss in my third pregnancy. By then I expected to miscarry.

After I saw a reproductive endocrinologist for testing and treatment of what turned out to be low progesterone levels and blood-clotting factors, I had two successful pregnancies, but the memory of my miscarriages remains with me.

Some Basic Facts About Miscarriage

In case your practitioner hasn't already given you this information, let's review the basics. According to the Mayo Clinic, the term *miscarriage* refers to the loss of a pregnancy before 20 weeks, and 10 to 20 percent of known pregnancies end in miscarriage. (A loss after 20 weeks is called a stillbirth.) An even higher number of pregnancies may end in miscarriage before a woman even knows she is pregnant. About 80 percent of confirmed miscarriages occur in the first trimester—or before the twelfth week in the traditional 40-week dating system.

In the overwhelming majority of cases, no one knows why miscarriage occurs. Most studies of possible miscarriage causes have concluded that the actions of the mother and her partner have nothing to do with the pregnancy loss.

One study found that the risk of miscarriage varied according to a woman's reproductive history. In the study, 5 percent of confirmed first pregnancies, and first pregnancies after live births, ended in miscarriage. For women who had had one miscarriage, the risk of having another was 20 percent. After two miscarriages, the risk of another was 28 percent, and after three miscarriages the risk of another loss was 43 percent.

Most practitioners agree that after three miscarriages testing for known triggers is prudent, and many practitioners will run tests for women who have had two losses rather than wait for a third. This makes sense, because the odds of finding potentially treatable abnormalities are approximately the same after two or three consecutive losses. Many insurance companies, however, define recurrent miscarriage as three or more consecutive losses, and so refuse to pay for tests after two losses. Since the tests can cost thousands of dollars, many women must undergo a third miscarriage before they can receive a medical evaluation.

In cases of recurrent miscarriage, a treatable cause can be found about 60 percent of the time. But a study of women who had had multiple miscarriages for which tests determined no causes showed that nearly 70 percent of these women eventually had successful pregnancies. So you should know that the chances are always in your favor that you will have a baby someday, although this may not be comforting to you while you are grieving.

Bleeding in pregnancy does not necessarily indicate a miscarriage. The diagnostic process involves ultrasound tests, serial blood tests for the pregnancy hormone hCG (human chorionic gonadotropin), or both of these. An ultrasound test, usually vaginal, can be used to assess a baby's development as early as the fifth week of gestation, when the gestational sac—the sac in which the baby develops—becomes visible. At approximately seven weeks, depending on the ultrasound machine used, the baby's heartbeat becomes visible (a vaginal ultrasound can detect a heartbeat earlier than an abdominal ultrasound).

The ultrasound can be used to diagnose miscarriage in a number of ways. If the hCG level in a blood test indicates that a yolk sac or heartbeat ought to be visible, and a vaginal ultrasound fails to show this level of development, miscarriage is likely. If the baby appears less developed than the dates of the last menstrual period and a positive pregnancy test would indicate (if, for example, a woman confirmed she was pregnant at four weeks after the start of her last menstrual period, and then an ultrasound a month later measured the pregnancy at only five weeks), then a miscarriage is likely. If two ultrasounds taken a week apart show no growth, then miscarriage can be diagnosed. Whenever a heartbeat is visible on one ultrasound scan but not detected on a subsequent scan, pregnancy loss has most likely occurred.

In early pregnancy, blood hCG levels normally rise continuously and should roughly double every two to three days. If the hCG level falls from one test to the next, miscarriage is almost certain. Levels that rise slowly but do not double over a period of at least three days are indicative of a possible problem but not necessarily of pregnancy loss. One study found that some women whose hCG levels rose as little as 53 percent in two days turned out to have viable pregnancies. Slowly rising hCG levels can, however, indicate an ectopic pregnancy (a pregnancy not in the uterus; see page 8). Because an ectopic pregnancy can endanger a woman's life, a doctor will closely monitor any pregnancy in which hCG levels rise slowly.

Because the hCG doubling time normally lengthens as pregnancy progresses, the pregnancy must be accurately dated if serial hCG levels are to be a reliable miscarriage indicator. After about seven weeks' gestation (five weeks after conception and about three weeks after the first missed period, assuming a 28-day cycle), an ultrasound scan is a more reliable way to test for viability.

Blood tests are the only means of checking whether hCG is rising properly. Some women try to monitor their hCG levels by repeatedly testing their urine with home pregnancy test kits. They expect the line on the stick to darken over time, and if it instead gets lighter they fear the worst. Because the concentration of hCG in your urine will vary quite a lot depending on the time of day, how much liquid you have had to drink, and other factors, urine tests are not an accurate means of judging how your hCG levels are rising, and attempting to check your levels in this way might cause you unnecessary stress.

A woman's body does not recognize immediately that a pregnancy is not viable. Even after an exam indicates a likely miscarriage, six weeks or more may pass before bleeding begins. This is one reason many women opt for the procedure known as dilation and curettage, or D&C, after tests indicate a pregnancy loss (see pages 8 and 13).

A Quick Guide to Miscarriage Terms

Many practitioners don't use the term *miscarriage;* instead they opt for the more clinical-sounding *spontaneous abortion.* This term, which refers to the natural loss of a baby during the first trimester or the first part of the second trimester, is not to be confused with the term *induced abortion,* which refers to the elective ending of a pregnancy. Even if the practitioner carefully avoids the word abortion, it is likely to appear on billing and insurance statements following a miscarriage. Some women find this very upsetting.

> *To me the term* spontaneous abortion *implies that you chose to miscarry.*
>
> —WANDA

> *I saw that my chart said "habitual abortion." I know it is just a medical term, but it still hurts, for some reason, to see it in writing.*
>
> —ASTRID

The first time I saw the words spontaneous abortion, *they were on the bill from my first miscarriage. I called the doctor's office and said I had not had an abortion. I did find it offensive.*

—BETH

When I was pregnant again after the first miscarriage, I read the words spontaneous abortion *in my records while waiting for my doctor to come in. Those words broke my heart.*

—TAMMIE

I will not use the term *spontaneous abortion* in this book beyond this section. At the time of my own miscarriages, I found myself cringing every time I heard the word *abortion* applied to what I was going through, especially when the clerk in the clinic where I was having my D&C after my second miscarriage mistook the diagnosis "missed abortion" as meaning an elective abortion gone awry.

Unfortunately, *spontaneous abortion* is not the only difficult term you may hear. Here is a list of some of the most common medical terms that may have come up during your experience. (You will find some less common terms in the glossary at the end of the book.)

Aneuploidy. In this type of chromosomal abnormality, a baby has either a missing chromosome or one more than is normal.

Biochemical pregnancy. You may have heard this term—or *chemical pregnancy,* which means the same—if you had a very early miscarriage that happened shortly after you found out you were pregnant. Being diagnosed as having had a biochemical pregnancy doesn't mean that you weren't really pregnant. Rather, it means that blood and urine tests for hCG are the only evidence of the pregnancy; the fertilized egg never developed to the point that its existence could be confirmed by ultrasound (pregnancies confirmed by nonchemical means such as ultrasound are considered "clinical" pregnancies). In a biochemical pregnancy, a sperm and egg meet, and conception occurs, but the egg does not implant properly in the uterus. A woman experiencing a biochemical pregnancy may get a faint positive on a home pregnancy test and then start to bleed a day or two later.

Women who are not actively trying to conceive and not keeping close tabs on their menstrual cycles may easily have biochemical pregnancies and never realize it. For this reason, we don't know how often biochemical pregnancies occur in the general population. You may read that as many as 70 to 80 percent of pregnancies end in loss; these figures reflect high estimates of the rate of biochemical pregnancy. Practitioners often advise women to wait until their period is several days late before taking a pregnancy test so that they might avoid grief over a biochemical pregnancy.

Blighted ovum. When an ovum is blighted, the baby stops developing at a very early stage and disintegrates. The mother's body fails to recognize the loss, and the gestational sac may continue to grow. The mother may continue to experience pregnancy symptoms, and the loss of the baby may not be detected until 10 to 12 weeks along, when an ultrasound test shows an empty gestational sac. Sometimes a blighted ovum must be cleared with a D&C.

Chromosomal abnormality. This term indicates that the developing baby has the wrong number of chromosomes or some type of translocation in the chromosomes (see chapter 2). Babies with chromosomal abnormalities are often miscarried because the abnormalities are incompatible with life; in fact, chromosomal abnormalities are thought to be the most common cause of miscarriage. Some chromosomal abnormalities, such as Down syndrome, do not prevent a baby's survival through a full term of pregnancy and beyond.

D&C (dilation and curettage). When a woman has a missed or incomplete miscarriage, or she has started bleeding and does not wish to wait for the process to finish naturally, a D&C is an option. If a woman is experiencing a hemorrhage or is at high risk of infection because of tissue remaining in her uterus, a D&C may be a necessity. In a D&C, the physician scrapes or vacuums out the tissue that remains in the uterus.

Ectopic pregnancy. This refers to a pregnancy in which the embryo has implanted somewhere outside the uterus, usually in one of the fallopian tubes. Ectopic pregnancies either miscarry naturally or require termination to preserve the woman's health. Ectopic pregnancies are not viable.

If they develop for too long, they can result in internal hemorrhage, rupture and possibly loss of a fallopian tube, and death.

Embryo. This term refers to the developing baby from the fourth through the eighth week of pregnancy.

Fetal demise. This term can refer to any pregnancy that is lost after 10 weeks.

Fetal pole. In the early stages of pregnancy, practitioners sometimes refer to the tiny developing baby as a "fetal pole," particularly when they are analyzing ultrasound images. The fetal pole should be visible by six weeks in an ultrasound test.

Gestational sac. This is the sac, implanted in the uterus, in which the baby develops. It should be visible within the womb in an ultrasound test by the middle of the fifth week of pregnancy.

Habitual abortion. Although this sounds like a habit of obtaining elective abortions, this term actually refers to a woman who has had two or more miscarriages. A better term, obviously, is *recurrent miscarriage.*

hCG (human chorionic gonadotropin). This hormone, if present in your blood or urine, indicates that you are pregnant. It is what causes the second line to appear in home pregnancy tests. Tests for hCG can also indicate a probable miscarriage, if two blood draws taken two to three days apart fail to show a normal rise in the concentration of the hormone.

Incomplete miscarriage/abortion. This term is used when a woman's body has not passed all of the tissue from a miscarried pregnancy. Tissue retained in the uterus can cause continued bleeding and pose a risk of infection. If tissue is retained too long as determined by a doctor, a D&C (dilation and curettage; see page 8) is usually recommended.

Misoprostol. This medication is sometimes used to speed up an incomplete or missed miscarriage for women who wish to avoid a D&C but do not want to wait out a natural miscarriage.

Missed miscarriage/abortion. This refers to a pregnancy that has been diagnosed as unviable, through an ultrasound scan, before bleeding has begun. Some cases of missed miscarriages are due to blighted ova (see page 8).

Molar pregnancy (gestational trophoblastic disease). This terrible type of loss results from a problem during fertilization. Upon implantation, an abnormal placenta grows instead of a baby. In a **partial molar pregnancy**, a baby may form, but with too many chromosomes to sustain life. A molar pregnancy can be a medical emergency; in rare cases, the abnormal placenta may behave like a cancerous tumor and threaten the woman's health. Extremely high hCG levels sometimes indicate a molar pregnancy. Before trying for a new pregnancy, women who have had molar pregnancies need careful medical monitoring to make sure that their hCG levels have gone down completely and remained low for a period of time.

Progesterone. This is another hormone produced at high levels during pregnancy. Progesterone stimulates the body to support the pregnancy, by relaxing the uterus, stimulating the development of breast tissue, maintaining the early placenta, and more. Low progesterone levels are associated with miscarriages, but practitioners disagree about whether low levels of this hormone are a cause or an effect of an impending miscarriage. Read more about progesterone in chapter 3.

Spontaneous abortion. This term refers to a miscarriage, or the nonelective ending of a pregnancy before 20 weeks.

Stillbirth. The loss of a pregnancy after 20 weeks.

Threatened miscarriage/abortion. This term refers to any unexpected first- or second-trimester bleeding. About 20 percent of all pregnant women experience a threatened miscarriage, and about 30 percent of these women go on to miscarry.

Triploidy. This is an abnormality in which a baby has three complete sets of chromosomes.

Trisomy. In this form of aneuploidy, a baby has three copies of one chromosome. Down syndrome results from trisomy of chromosome 21.

Venipuncture. You may see this term appear on a lab bill. It just means the drawing of blood for blood tests.

Yolk sac. This component of a very early developing embryo should be visible in an ultrasound test by about five weeks.

Zygote. This term for the developing baby refers to the period from conception until the fourth week of gestation.

It's Okay to Grieve

Let's make one thing clear right now: It's perfectly healthy and normal to grieve the loss of your baby. People may say, "There was probably something wrong with it" or "It was for the best." Although such comments are hurtful, people who make them usually are well intentioned; they may just not know what to say and most likely do not understand that what they are saying does not help you. Do not let anyone make you feel like you're wrong to be sad for having lost your baby. Suppressing your grief will only make you feel worse in the long run and delay healing. Unresolved grief can pop up at the least expected moments, and scientists are only beginning to understand all the effects that such stress can have on the body.

> *The doc said I had nothing to worry about; since there was a strong, healthy heartbeat I had only a 5 percent chance of miscarriage. We went home elated. Two days later I started passing very large clots. I went to the emergency room and was told that my hCG levels had fallen from 3,500 to 2,900. They wanted to do a D&C right away.*
>
> —HEATHER

> *The morning when we found out that I was going to miscarry, I felt numb, as if I were having a bad dream. It was as if I were outside my own body looking in. I felt the most pain for our baby, Cole, knowing that soon his heart was going to stop on its own. That morning he still had a heartbeat. By 5:30 p.m. it had stopped.*
>
> —JODY

> *I went to the ER for my second miscarriage. None of the ER docs knew what to do with me. One of them gave me a blood pregnancy test and excitedly told me it was positive so I must be okay. I had to explain to him—a medical professional!—that I would have a positive pregnancy test even if I were in the process of miscarrying the*

baby. I demanded and got an ultrasound, but the technician refused to tell me if she saw the baby or not. She said someone else had to read the results. I became hysterical, and she finally told me not to tell anyone that she had told me but she did see the baby and it looked okay. They sent me home, and I lost the baby shortly after walking in my front door.

—FRIEDA

That night was possibly the worst night of my life. I felt as if I was going into labor. My partner was out, and my two-and-a-half-year-old daughter was asleep. I was exhausted but could not sleep, and the pain was horrific. I called the hospital; the nurse told me to take painkillers and that if things got worse I would have to go to the emergency room. At about 11:30 P.M., I telephoned my good friend and neighbor, and she came over and gave me a much-needed hug. After I sobbed for an hour my partner walked in. I went to bed, and my neighbor went home.

—MEREDITH

I went to the ER with the third loss. There was a six-hour wait, and there were women in there crying, obviously going through the same thing I was. Some couples were coming out of examining rooms holding ultrasound scan photos and beaming; the babies had been checked and found to be okay. I had to give my details three times to different staff members. A doctor checked me over and sent me for an ultrasound scan, which confirmed my fears. I then had to sit in a quiet room by myself until my husband arrived and we decided what to do.

—SARAH

If Your Miscarriage Isn't Yet Complete

Many women head to the emergency room if they experience any bleeding in pregnancy. Trying to get help this way is time-consuming, stressful, and usually unnecessary. Unless you are in severe pain, it may be best to call your practitioner's office before heading to the hospital, even in the middle of the night. Usually, an obstetrical-gynecological practice will have someone on call who can answer your questions, and staying home until the morning will probably not affect the viability of the pregnancy. Emergency-room doctors will probably not be able to do anything for you even if you are miscarrying. To reliably diagnose a miscarriage, you need two separate hCG tests, two or more days apart, or an ultrasound scan to determine whether a heartbeat is visible. The emergency-room doctor may do the ultrasound for you, but, if you're less than seven to eight weeks along or not entirely sure of your dates, a single scan may not be reliable in diagnosing or ruling out miscarriage. The experience of going to the emergency room may be an added stress that you just don't need.

The D&C Question

If you've not yet fully miscarried at the time you pick up this book but have received the news of an impending miscarriage, your practitioner may have brought up the question of a D&C. Routine D&Cs upon detection of miscarriage have become a common practice among many obstetrician-gynecologists.

In some situations, a D&C is a medical necessity. If you're hemorrhaging or you have been diagnosed with an incomplete miscarriage—that is, your body is retaining tissue for too long, posing a risk of infection—your practitioner will let you know that a D&C is necessary. A D&C may also be necessary if the miscarriage happens under circumstances in which the practitioner feels it's medically unlikely that you will be able to miscarry naturally.

Sometimes a D&C is not medically necessary. If a D&C is presented as optional rather than essential, you may not be sure what to do. In the event that the procedure is not necessary for your physical health, here are some things to keep in mind when making this choice:

REASONS TO HAVE A D&C

* A D&C speeds up the process of miscarriage. After you learn of your baby's loss, the miscarriage may take hours or weeks to complete nat-

urally. Once bleeding begins, it will probably be over within two weeks, but the wait may be much longer if the bleeding has yet to begin. Many women prefer to have a D&C just to have the physical part over with so they can move on with grieving and accepting the loss.

- If you have a D&C, it may be possible to have tests done afterward that may determine the cause of the loss. If this is your first miscarriage, your practitioner may not offer tests, but if you have had two or more miscarriages, testing might be an option. Genetic tests can either confirm or rule out chromosomal anomalies as a cause of your miscarriages, and this may be helpful when you decide whether and how to proceed with treatment. These tests are expensive, however—they can cost more than $1,000—and your health insurance may not cover them. Some parents are uncomfortable with the idea of genetically testing a miscarried baby regardless of the cost.

- With a D&C, you won't have to see what comes out, as you might in a natural miscarriage. If you are put under general anesthesia for the D&C, as some women prefer, you won't be awake for the procedure at all. General anesthesia involves more risks than local anesthesia, however, so you may prefer to use the latter, and so may your physician. Most D&Cs today are done with conscious sedation. Address any questions about anesthesia to your doctor.

- You may experience less intense physical pain with a D&C. Some women who miscarry the natural way experience heavy cramping. After a D&C, the physical pain is often of shorter duration and less intense. This varies with the individual, however. Sometimes recovery from a D&C is more painful than the typical natural miscarriage.

- At least one study has found that women who miscarry naturally have a higher rate of subsequent hospital admissions than do women who have had D&Cs.

REASONS *NOT* TO HAVE A D&C

- The procedure can be something of an ordeal. Although an overnight stay is usually unnecessary, you will probably have to check into the hospital and go through preparatory tests. Sometimes, however, a D&C is done in the doctor's office or in the emergency room.

- The procedure is invasive. You will likely experience some strong emotions before and after the operation, and the clinical environment might make you more uneasy. Just as some women cannot handle the idea of continuing a pregnancy that will not result in a live baby, others cannot handle the psychological ramifications of a D&C. For many women, the idea of a D&C just feels wrong. They are more comfortable with letting nature take its course.

- A D&C is not risk-free. Complications are not common, but neither are they rare. Potential risks include a punctured uterus or other scarring. Also, sometimes the procedure fails to remove all the tissue and has to be repeated. Anesthesia, especially general anesthesia, carries some risks. Be sure to discuss any concerns about risks with your doctor.

Deciding whether or not to have D&C is not easy, and the decision is very, very personal. You and your partner need to decide according to what feels right for you given your individual circumstances.

I had an ultrasound and saw the dead baby, and then we organized the D&C in two days' time. The next day my partner and I woke up and cried, and I felt like a part of me had been taken away. We were very sad all day and did not want to leave the house and face the public. The day of the D&C I felt okay.

—TAYA

When I woke up from the D&C, I felt relieved knowing that it was all over (except for the spotting during the recovery period, which I had been advised about) and that I didn't have to suffer while waiting for the natural loss to occur.

—MEGHAN

Author's Story

I opted for a D&C following my second miscarriage. I was almost 10 weeks along, but the baby, according to an ultrasound scan, had stopped growing at six weeks. Nervous and worried, I had been spotting for about four days when the clots began to come out and the miscarriage was confirmed. I couldn't sleep. I couldn't focus on my work. And nothing on earth could make me smile. The days passed torturously. I needed the experience to be over with so I could move on.

I was scheduled to have the D&C at noon. That day, the phone woke me at 6:00 A.M. A nurse from the hospital asked me to come in right away, because the doctor had to perform a cesarean section that afternoon and wanted to get my operation over with early to avoid having to move a lot of equipment in a hurry. I said I could *not* come in right away; I would be in at noon as scheduled.

When I arrived at the hospital, I changed into a gown in a room in which several people were recuperating from surgery. My husband waited with me for about 20 minutes, until an orderly arrived to wheel me into the operating room. An anesthesiologist came in to talk about choices in sedation. I told him that I wanted to be asleep and I didn't want to remember anything.

The next thing I remember is waking up in the recovery room. My husband was brought in to talk to me soon thereafter, and the nurse informed me that my doctor had left me a prescription for pain medication. I was woozy for a few hours, but medication couldn't help what hurt the most. My husband and I went out for Chinese food. The waitress, seeing the Band-Aid on my arm from the IV line and apparently thinking I'd had a routine blood test, asked if I was pregnant. We overheard a couple bragging about their twins who would be born soon.

I don't remember any other details, but I think I cried most of the rest of the day. The next morning I woke up feeling as if I'd been run over by a truck. I needed the pain medication, but there was no bleeding. I felt back to normal physically within a few days, and my period returned after eight weeks.

I've had two natural miscarriages at home, and they were messy. I had to deal with them all by myself. When I had my D&C, it was nice to go to sleep and let someone else take care of me.

—PAULA

I was really upset about the idea of having a D&C, because I knew I wasn't going to be able to hold or see anything of this child. Also, I felt like it was a drive-through kind of thing; one minute you are pregnant, and the next minute you're not.

—MARTINA

I wasn't allowed to have my husband or anyone there with me, and although they gave me a little pain medicine I felt like my insides were being scraped away. After the procedure I was given a pamphlet on baby loss and a paper to fill out about my feelings over what had just happened. I asked if I could have a burial for my baby, and they said this was not something they allowed. I asked what they would do with my baby, and the nurse nonchalantly said, "Oh, we just get rid of them in the incinerator." I was so hurt, but didn't know how to stick up for myself or for the baby I lost. Sometimes it still haunts me.

—OKSANA

I felt a nagging concern that maybe the baby was really alive and I was somehow killing it. Some of the staff at the hospital were totally unsympathetic; they treated my D&C like a tooth extraction.

—NANCY

After having a D&C, many women want to see the baby, or at least know where the baby is. The baby and placenta are usually sent to a lab for pathological examination immediately after the procedure. With a late loss, you may be able to have a picture taken of the baby and even keep a lock of hair. With an early-pregnancy loss, however, the baby, sac, and placenta are usually smaller than an inch and indistinguishable. In this case, there is no recognizable baby to hold or bury.

After a D&C, you will probably experience bleeding or spotting for 5 to 14 days, although the time may be longer or shorter than this. Please check with your doctor if you are concerned about heavy bleeding or pain after a D&C. After the procedure, your hCG level should continue to fall, and your pregnancy symptoms should begin to diminish. You will probably return to having normal monthly cycles within two to three months. Your physician may advise you to wait until you have had a normal period or two before trying to get pregnant again (see chapter 6).

A NOTE ON MISDIAGNOSED
MISCARRIAGES AND D&CS

Very rarely, a miscarriage is misdiagnosed. This sometimes happens when a woman goes to the emergency room, usually when around six weeks pregnant, with bleeding and cramping. The practitioner does an ultrasound test, sees no gestational sac and no fetal heartbeat, and, judging from the date the woman's last menstrual period started, concludes that the woman is miscarrying and suggests an immediate D&C. In such a case, the practitioner has assumed that the woman knew exactly when her last period started and that she ovulated on day 14 of her cycle. In fact, a deviation of even a few days from either of these dates could mean the baby's heartbeat wouldn't yet be visible on the ultrasound machine, especially if abdominal rather than vaginal ultrasound was used.

Many women do not have regular 28-day cycles. If a woman ovulates on day 21, for example, the fetal heartbeat might not be visible six weeks after the first day of the last menstrual period, because this would be only three weeks after conception. In this case, the baby should show development typical at five weeks of pregnancy, not six. This is why many doctors will not diagnose a miscarriage from a single ultrasound scan without other data indicating the gestational age, such as hCG tests. If the baby does not show expected signs of development and the gestational age is uncertain, the doctor will tell the mother to come back in a week for another test. This wait will be an anxious one for the mother, but most doctors want to avoid suggesting a D&C or diagnosing a miscarriage until they are certain that the pregnancy is not viable.

The likelihood of a miscarriage misdiagnosis is exceedingly small. Occasionally, however, it happens, and a D&C is performed prematurely. If your baby shows no heartbeat and you have any doubt about whether he should be developed enough to show one, it may be wise to wait a few extra days before deciding on a D&C.

Nonsurgical Miscarriages

If after learning of an impending miscarriage you decide to wait for nature to take its course, the process could begin immediately or days or weeks later. It is impossible to predict the length of the wait. In the meantime, you may experience morning sickness or other pregnancy symptoms despite falling hCG levels or the lack of a heartbeat on the ultrasound. The wait can be very difficult emotionally. Many women are not able to tolerate feeling pregnant when they know that a miscarriage is inevitable but don't know when the process will begin or end. Others prefer to wait and let the pregnancy end naturally rather than have an invasive D&C.

Another option for women who wish to avoid a D&C is what's called a "medically assisted" or "medically managed" miscarriage. (A miscarriage completed with a D&C is called a "surgically managed" miscarriage; allowing a miscarriage to occur with no interventions is called "expectant management.") Some physicians are now prescribing drugs, such as misoprostol, to speed up a miscarriage when the diagnosis is certain. The availability of medically managed miscarriage varies by practitioner, and not all physicians offer it to their patients. It is often a very painful experience that continues for several days.

With any nonsurgical miscarriage that happens in the first trimester, you should expect bleeding that is somewhat heavier than you normally experience during a menstrual period and that is accompanied by cramping. You may see clots and clumps of tissue in the discharge. The further along you are in pregnancy, the more bleeding, pain, and visible tissue you can expect. Provided your miscarriage isn't accompanied by excessive bleeding—most practitioners define this as soaking through a sanitary pad every hour—or severe pain, you can probably get through the process at home and avoid the stress of the emergency room. Remember, emergency-room doctors cannot stop a first-trimester miscarriage in progress or prevent one that is impending; they can only ensure that your own health is not endangered. But if you have any worry at all that your bleeding is too heavy or that your pregnancy might be ectopic, head to the emergency room for treatment.

Most natural miscarriages do not happen all at once. Movies and fictional stories often depict a miscarriage as a sudden thing, when in truth it can be drawn out like a menstrual period. The bleeding may last for as long as two weeks, although it should not remain heavy for that long a time.

If your miscarriage happens very shortly after you learn you are pregnant, you may not notice anything but blood. But if you were six weeks along or further before the baby stopped growing, you may see a small gestational sac as well as numerous small blood clots or pieces of tissue. You may want to collect this material in a small plastic bag, store it in the refrigerator if this happens at night, and take it to your practitioner's office the next day for examination. If the baby stopped growing at more than eight weeks' gestation, you may pass the remains of a recognizable baby. This may understandably be traumatic. You may want to save the tissue and have some kind of burial.

If you have had more than one loss, you may want to save some of the tissue for chromosomal analysis. One way to do this is to place a sieve over the toilet. If this is more than you can handle emotionally, though, it's okay; you're only human.

The severity of pain during a natural miscarriage varies from woman to woman. If your miscarriage happens very early in your pregnancy, you

---

If You Are Rh-Negative

If you are among the 10 percent or so of people who do not carry the blood protein called the Rh factor, you should be given an injection of Rh immune globulin (RhoGAM) within 72 hours of your D&C or the start of your bleeding. This will minimize the risk that the baby's blood, if Rh-positive, will trigger an antibody reaction in your body. If you were to have such a reaction, your immune response in a subsequent pregnancy could seriously threaten the baby's health. The odds of Rh sensitization with a first-trimester loss are low, but most practitioners give the shot as a precaution.

Author's Story

*M*y first and third miscarriages happened naturally. The first occurred at only five weeks' gestation and was virtually indistinguishable from a menstrual period except that I bled for just over a week instead of my normal five or six days. In the third, I was six weeks along when I learned through ultrasound and hCG blood tests that the gestational sac was far too small to be viable. After the ultrasound, I was angry at my doctor because she had told me my hCG levels were fine after they had doubled between two blood tests. She had thought that the tests were taken two days apart, when they had actually been two weeks apart, and I was the one who had to point that out to her. Unfortunately, such errors are a common experience among women undergoing miscarriage and are indicative of the less than optimal care that women in this country receive in such situations.

I didn't want to go through another D&C. A D&C had seemed appropriate after my second miscarriage. Now I was fatalistic; even before the slow-rising hCG levels were identified, I had almost expected my pregnancy to end in miscarriage. So I chose to experience the loss naturally at home.

The sac was very tiny, whitish, and translucent. The baby had stopped growing at just five or six weeks, so the sac was perhaps the size of a pea, and nothing was visible inside. I wasn't sure what it was when I saw it, and I wasn't thinking totally clearly, so I threw it away. Only later did I realize what it was. I will never forget the sight of it, and the memory of throwing it in the trash still haunts me sometimes.

will probably feel little more pain than you do in a regular menstrual period. If you are further along than six weeks, you may have some heavy cramping, and you should be sure to give yourself time to rest. Ask your practitioner to recommend a painkiller in the event that your cramping becomes too severe. Don't try to be a superwoman; you're suffering enough already. Stay in bed for a few days, eat your favorite ice cream, and ask your partner to rent a pile of movies (but warn him not to bring home anything that involves pregnancy or babies).

If you are taking misoprostol or another medication to speed up your miscarriage, the process should be much like a natural miscarriage. But please check with your practitioner regarding what is normal, what is not, and when to seek additional treatment.

Ectopic Pregnancies

Ectopic pregnancies, or pregnancies that occur outside the uterus (usually in one of the fallopian tubes), often get overlooked in discussion of miscarriages. This is unfortunate, because they are common: They happen in 1 out of every 40 to 100 pregnancies. The risk of ectopic pregnancy is higher in women who have had a tubal ligation reversed, who have conceived while using an IUD, who have pelvic inflammatory disease, or who have become pregnant through in vitro fertilization. An ectopic pregnancy may occur when scar tissue or a structural problem with a fallopian tube prevents the egg from reaching the uterus. Like other pregnancy losses, it may also occur randomly, in the absence of any known risk factor.

Symptoms of ectopic pregnancy vary. Sometimes hCG levels rise normally, and sometimes they do not. An ectopic pregnancy may be diagnosed after hCG levels fail to rise properly, or when the hCG levels are at a point that the pregnancy should be visible in an ultrasound scan of the uterus, but is not. Using ultrasound, the practitioner detects the pregnancy in the tube or assumes it is located elsewhere, where the ultrasound can't detect it. Sometimes the woman reports pain on one side of her abdomen.

If the embryo is not growing and not developing in a way that threatens the tube, no treatment may be necessary. But many ectopic pregnancies are medical emergencies. If the baby is growing in the fallopian tube as if it were implanted normally in the uterus, the fallopian tube can rupture. Such rupture can be fatal to the mother as well as the baby.

A diagnosed ectopic pregnancy is managed in one of three ways, depending on the woman's preference and the risk posed to her health. If the gestational sac remains small, the hCG levels are lower than 1,000, and the hCG levels are falling rather than rising, the woman may be given the option of waiting to miscarry with no intervention. For an ectopic pregnancy in which the mother does not appear to be in the process of miscarrying naturally and in which rupture is not imminent, the woman may be given the medication methotrexate to induce miscarriage. This approach works 87 to 95 percent of the time and avoids surgery. If the physician deems the ectopic pregnancy to be a medical emergency—if, for example, the gestational sac has grown too large and is threatening to cause tubal rupture, or if the woman has had pain for longer than 24 hours or is suffering other symptoms—surgery may be recommended. In the event of an actual tubal rupture, immediate surgery is required.

If you have experienced an ectopic pregnancy and have had to terminate the life of a desired baby to save your own, you may feel guilt as well as grief. This is natural, even though you know there was no chance of the pregnancy continuing to term.

Couples who experience ectopic pregnancies may be even more likely to suffer insensitive comments from friends and relatives. Because of the potential danger to a woman's life, you may hear comments like "Just be glad they caught it in time" instead of "I'm so sorry for your loss." Unfortunately, people sometimes forget in their concern for the mother that the couple also lost a child.

Following an ectopic pregnancy, you may be worried about your ability to conceive again. Please talk to your practitioner about whether you need to be evaluated for scar tissue or endometriosis that may have contributed to or resulted from the ectopic pregnancy. If you had a fallopian tube removed to prevent a rupture, or if your tube ruptured and could not be repaired, your ability to conceive may be reduced. Eighty-five percent of women who have had an ectopic pregnancy can go on to have a full-term pregnancy, but repeat cases of ectopic pregnancy occur 10 to 20 percent of the time, so your practitioner will probably want you to have an early checkup the next time you get pregnant to make sure that the baby is implanted where it should be.

Gestational Trophoblastic Disease

If you are reading this after being diagnosed with the rare condition called gestational trophoblastic disease, or molar pregnancy, my heart goes out to you. A molar pregnancy results when a sperm fertilizes an egg that has no nucleus, or when two sperm fertilize a single egg. The mass in the uterus, which can never become a live baby, is called a hydatidiform mole. In some cases, molar cells can invade the lining of the uterus and become cancerous.

If you have had a molar pregnancy, you may be experiencing any number of feelings, and, as with women who have had ectopic pregnancies, your friends and relatives may overlook the fact that you're recovering from a pregnancy loss and the grief that accompanies it. In the coming weeks, you may wish to seek out a support group dedicated to this condition. You will probably need to have a D&C and then weekly blood tests to make sure your hCG levels return to zero, and your practitioner will probably tell you to wait six months or a year before conceiving again. This way your practitioner will be able to make sure that the molar pregnancy has not become cancerous and to distinguish residual hCG from the molar pregnancy from hCG produced by a new pregnancy.

What You're Feeling

Chapter 5 discusses coping with miscarriage in depth, but at this point you should know that there are as many ways of reacting to miscarriage as there are people who miscarry. Some women aren't much bothered by their miscarriages, for any number of reasons, and that's perfectly valid. Others are crushed and struggle to cope with the experience, and that's also perfectly valid. Since you are reading this book, you are likely in the latter category.

Your experience may have left you feeling detached and numb, barely able to believe what happened or to care about anything in your life, or you may have a tremendous sadness that feels like it's never going to go away. You may be alternating between the two, or you may fall somewhere in between. If your miscarriage has happened within the past several days, you are dealing with a hormonal crash that may intensify your sadness. Whatever you're feeling, it is probably normal. You need to give yourself time to grieve. The loss will always be a part of you, but you can trust that it won't always feel as overwhelming as it does in the beginning. Chapter 5 will help you find ways to cope.

It's not enough to say I was shocked. It was like being both a spectator to and actress in a slow-motion horror movie.

—JESSIE

My world crumbled. You build up your love for this little person whom you have never seen, only to find out there is no heartbeat. I was angry at God for bringing my pregnancy this far only to take it away, but most of all I was angry at myself because I couldn't carry a child full term.

—TAMMY

The first miscarriage was devastating. After the other three, I was surprisingly numb, as if miscarriage was beginning to be a habit or routine. I think that I just could not possibly feel any more pain.

—JILL

When I found out I was pregnant for the first time after eight years of trying, it was as if I had been given the greatest gift possible. Then it was taken from me so quickly that I felt like the victim of a mean joke.

—MICHELLE

I didn't think a miscarriage could ever happen to me; it's something horrible that happens to other people. I lay on the couch and cried the entire weekend. I still think about it almost every day, even though I am trying to keep a positive attitude, especially since we have started trying to conceive again.

—EMILY

The first time I miscarried, I was in shock. The second time was worse; I never in a million years thought it would happen a second time, and I went into a deep depression. The third time I cried, "Why is this happening again? Why me?" I fell into an even worse depression than with the second miscarriage.

—JOCELYN

There were days I didn't want to talk to anyone; there were days I never stopped crying; there were days I was so angry at God I thought I would never find peace again. I took a week off work after each miscarriage. I could barely get myself up to take a shower.

—TAMMY

We started to clean our house even though it was already clean. My mom came over to be with us, and I just remember my husband vacuuming while I was cleaning the spare room. We were certainly in shock.

—JODY

We held each other and cried for a long time. We don't have other children, and we have been trying for over six years, so this loss was like a slap across the face.

—KIMBERLY

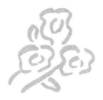

CHAPTER 2

Looking for Causes
of Miscarriage

ONCE YOU'RE OVER THE INITIAL SHOCK of your miscarriage, you will probably have one major question weighing on your mind: Why did this happen to me?

This chapter will focus on the causes of miscarriage. We will examine the research and consider both what is known about miscarriages and what is not known. We'll also look at some theories that haven't been proven yet about why miscarriages happen.

Some of the causes of miscarriage do not currently have known treatments, and some treatments cover multiple causes. For more information on what to do about conditions that cause miscarriage, if you already know you have them, skip ahead to chapter 3.

If you have had just one miscarriage, I won't tell you not to worry about having another. I hope you won't; the odds are that you won't. But I know that hearing and reading this over and over can be either reassuring or annoying. You may want to know exactly what happened to you and why. Because miscarriage is very common, and because a great many miscarriages result from random chromosomal abnormalities or one-time problems that will not happen again, your practitioner has probably advised you simply to try again. Although in a perfect world doctors might run a full set of tests after a first loss or even as a standard preconception checkup, just to catch that one woman in a dozen or so with a problem that could cause recurrent miscarriage, most practitioners will not order tests for causes of first-trimester losses until a woman has had at least two. (If your loss took place in the second trimester, your doctor may be willing to do a few tests, primarily for blood-clotting abnormalities.)

According to the American College of Obstetricians and Gynecologists, the frequency of abnormal findings is the same whether women are tested after two or three consecutive pregnancy losses. If you have had two or more consecutive miscarriages, therefore, your physician should be willing to perform tests for possible causes. If not, you'll want to find a physician who will. This book will help you come up with questions for your physician and get ready to take an active role in your care.

My intention is not to make you worry that you have a dozen things wrong with you. If reading too many details will make you do just that, I suggest looking first at the boxes throughout this chapter that summarize each condition. If you want to learn more, read the in-depth discussion that follows. If you want still more information, to read yourself or to show your doctor, see the relevant studies listed in the References at the end of the book. Search the Internet for each study by name, or visit the Web site for this book (www.aftermiscarriage.com) to find the abstracts.

Again, I am not a doctor. The information I'm providing here is intended to help you start a conversation with the person who *is* your medical practitioner.

For some people, thinking too much about possible causes of miscarriage just increases stress. The next time you get pregnant, you're going to worry regardless, but if reading about miscarriage causes will make you lie awake at night wondering if you have one of these problems, when in all likelihood you don't, you might read this chapter only through the section on chromosomal abnormalities and skip the sections on less common problems. Then you might go on to chapters 5 and 6, which discuss coping with the grief of miscarriage and getting ready to try again.

Searching for information on the Internet was confusing and often alarming. It seems that everything can contribute to the risk of miscarriage.

—Marlena

Online research made me feel less alone and helped me figure out what questions I should ask my doctor.

—WENDY

Sometimes my research was helpful, but mostly it just made me imagine that all kinds of crazy things were wrong with me.

—MICHELLE

For five years, I have researched online, in the library, and in my laboratory. I will not give up my relentless search for knowledge until I can understand why my miscarriage happened and how to prevent it from happening again. I find comfort in being able to match most doctors with my knowledge on the subject.

—LISA

Why Miscarriages Happen: In a Nutshell

As you know, an egg plus a sperm equals a fertilized egg, which travels down a woman's fallopian tube to implant in the uterus and then develop into a baby. But what you may not know is that a lot of other things are happening behind the scenes. A woman is born with her lifetime supply of eggs, but the chromosomes within the cells are not fully divided. Each month, starting at puberty, a small number of egg cells are activated, and one completes the process of cell division to result in a mature egg, which bursts from the ovary into one of the fallopian tubes about midway through the menstrual cycle. This is ovulation. If sperm are present in the tube or arrive within a day of ovulation, the egg can be fertilized. Sperm can persist as long as five days in the tube, but the numbers diminish over time. This is why you'll read that, when you're trying to conceive, you should have sex about every other day for the highest odds of conception.

Following fertilization, the egg drifts down the fallopian tube for about eight days before it implants in the uterus; at this point the hormone hCG (see page 187) is produced. HCG causes pregnancy tests to start showing positive within a few days after implantation (the exact timing of when a positive result will appear depends on the sensitivity of the test). The ovary begins producing progesterone, which stimulates the uterine lining to nourish the developing baby until the placenta is well developed and takes over progesterone production, around week 10 of the pregnancy, or eight weeks after conception.

Miscarriage results from some disruption to this process. If something goes wrong during cell division in the egg or the sperm that fertilizes it, the egg may carry the wrong number of chromosomes, and this may prevent it from developing into a baby (this is thought to be the most common cause of miscarriage). If a woman has a hormonal imbalance, this can also prevent the egg, or the uterine lining, from developing properly. If the fertilized egg implants in the fallopian tube or someplace else outside the uterus, an ectopic pregnancy results (see page 22). Immunological malfunctions may perhaps cause the woman's body to wrongly attack the developing baby (this is a topic of great controversy). Depending on where the egg implants, an abnormally shaped uterus may not be able to sustain the pregnancy. Any of these causes may be responsible for a single sporadic loss or for recurrent miscarriages.

Evaluating Information About Treatments for Miscarriage

If you talk with a few doctors, you'll hear differing opinions about miscarriage causes and treatment. You may hear everything from "Miscarriages are entirely preventable" to "There's nothing you can do, and you should learn to accept what you can't change."

The truth is somewhere in between. Some cases of recurrent miscarriage can be treated medically, and others cannot. Many studies suggest potential causes and even specific treatments but lack the large body of supporting medical literature that many physicians will require before pursuing treatment. Other potential causes are controversial; some studies support them, and other studies find no link between these suspected causes and miscarriage (differences in results may be due to differences in methodology). Still other causes and treatments may lack any supporting evidence but are trumpeted because theoretical models show they *might* work.

For these reasons, being an informed patient becomes key. You have to take a good look at the evidence yourself, decide what type of treatment you think you want (or don't want), and then find a practitioner whose philosophy matches your own. You may find one physician unwilling to pursue any treatment, and another who will throw everything but the kitchen sink at your problem.

Unlikely Causes of Miscarriage

Before we proceed with discussing miscarriage causes, let's consider factors that likely do *not* cause miscarriage. If you have been wondering about any of these, I hope this discussion will set your mind at ease.

Sex. Women commonly fear that sexual intercourse while pregnant could cause a miscarriage, but no one has ever found evidence that intercourse or orgasm has any bearing on whether a woman will miscarry.

Having a few drinks before finding out you are pregnant. A few studies have found links between miscarriage and consumption of small amounts of alcohol among women around the time of conception and even in male partners just before conception. Causation isn't certain, however. These studies may be confounded by unknown variables such as other lifestyle factors that coincide with alcohol consumption.

Moderate drinking (one to two drinks per day) and heavy drinking in the first trimester does increase miscarriage risk, but it's hard to draw any conclusions about the effects during the time before a woman knows she is pregnant. Usually, the embryo has been implanted in the uterus for only about a week when a woman discovers she is pregnant. For the first week following fertilization, the tiny developing ball of cells is merely floating in fluids and not sharing the mother's blood supply at all, and it seems unlikely that drinking alcohol would have any effect on the pregnancy during this period.

Using aspirin or another nonsteroidal anti-inflammatory drug before finding out that you are pregnant. Aspirin, ibuprofen, and other non-steroidal anti-inflammatory drugs (NSAIDs) are another gray area. It seems unlikely that using them in the immediate weeks after conception, when the embryo is floating in the fallopian tube or only very recently implanted, should pose a risk. Low-dose aspirin, in fact, is commonly used as part of the treatment protocol for miscarriages caused by blood-clotting disorders. Still, some studies have shown an association between the use of NSAIDs and miscarriage, although causation hasn't been established.

Acetaminophen (such as Tylenol) is generally considered a safe pain reliever for use in pregnancy, but check with your practitioner before taking it.

Lifting and other physical exertion. A few studies have correlated physical stress such as heavy lifting with increased miscarriage rates. Although the evidence is far from conclusive, it's probably best to avoid strenuous work when you are or may be pregnant. Mild to moderate exercise appears to pose no miscarriage risk.

Falling down in the first trimester. I have been unable to find any good studies about falling and miscarriages, but women who have fallen and then miscarried often worry that the fall caused the loss. The general consensus among doctors, however, is that a baby is well protected by amniotic fluid in the early stages of pregnancy and should be unaffected by falling or many other kinds of physical trauma.

Known Causes of Miscarriage

Factors that cause miscarriage fall into these categories:

* Chromosomal anomalies

* Infections

* Anatomical problems of the uterus

* Hormonal imbalances

* Blood-clotting disorders

* Immunological malfunctions

* Maternal illness

* Lifestyle factors

* Stress

Be forewarned that some of these conditions may be intertwined; one might be caused by another. Other causes of miscarriage may be yet unknown.

CHROMOSOMAL ANOMALIES

Chromosomal anomalies are considered the most common culprits in pregnancy loss. Many studies have concluded that about 60 percent of first-trimester pregnancy losses are caused by some type of chromosomal abnormality. Because this problem is so common, most practitioners assume that any woman's first miscarriage is probably due to random

Chromosomal anomalies at a glance

What are they? Errors in the number of chromosomes or re-arrangements of chromosomes in the developing baby.

Who is affected? Fifty to 60 percent of all miscarriages probably result from chromosomal anomalies. Usually, such an anomaly is a random occurrence, but in 3 to 5 percent of couples experiencing recurrent miscarriages either the male or the female is a carrier of a translocation (see page189). This means that the couple has at least a 50 percent risk of miscarriage with each pregnancy.

Why do some chromosomal anomalies cause miscarriage? Without the correct DNA for life, the baby cannot develop properly, or its development can be terminated by the mother's immune system, which may not recognize the baby as a baby because of the abnormal number of chromosomes.

What are the symptoms? The only way to tell if a miscarried baby had a chromosomal abnormality is to ask for a karyotype analysis of the fetal tissue, which will show the arrangement, number, size, shape, and other characteristics of the baby's chromosomes. A parent with a balanced translocation (see page 38) will probably show no outward symptoms, but recurrent miscarriage may be a symptom of a translocation in one or both of the parents.

How do I know if I have this problem? Karyotyping the tissue from a miscarriage will tell whether or not the cause of the miscarriage was chromosomal. Karyotyping the parents can determine whether either parent carries a translocation.

What can I do about this problem? No special treatment will prevent random chromosomal abnormalities, but couples who have one or more balanced translocations or who have experienced recurrent miscarriages caused by chromosomal abnormalities can consider preimplantation genetic diagnosis to improve the chances of a viable pregnancy in the future.

How certain is it that this problem causes miscarriages? Doctors are almost certain that chromosomal anomalies play a role in most miscarriages, although what causes the anomalies is less clear.

chromosomal abnormalities, and in fact the majority of women who have a single miscarriage will have a normal pregnancy the next time around. For this reason, few doctors run diagnostic tests after a first miscarriage, and many insurance companies won't pay the $500 to $800 cost of a chromosomal test. But the only way to know for sure that a loss is due to chromosomal anomalies is to have the embryo or fetus genetically tested (you may need to have a D&C in order to do this). The baby's complete set of chromosomes, or karyotype, can be examined for the most common anomalies that lead to miscarriage, such as aneuploidy or missing sections of chromosomes. If your baby's karyotype tests as abnormal, then you will know what caused the loss; if it tests as normal, you will know that you may find value in seeking further testing.

Some women cannot tolerate the idea of their babies, no matter how small, being sent to a lab for genetic testing. If you feel that a karyotype would be a violation of your baby's body, know that the choice is up to you. Although the information that a karyotype provides can be helpful, the results won't change what happened.

The test said "46XX"—a perfect girl; they told me they probably just ended up with a sample of my tissue.

—WENDY

If you proceed with a karyotype, be aware that you may not end up with a completely definitive answer regarding whether your loss was due to a chromosomal anomaly. Tissue removed during a D&C and sent for karyotyping may contain part of the decidua, or the lining of the pregnant uterus. If the embryo is missing or tiny, your tissue may grow instead of the baby's. Because karyotype tests performed after miscarriages often show a disproportionate number of 46XX (female) babies with normal chromosomes, many physicians consider karyotype results definitive only if the result shows a male baby or a female baby with clearly abnormal chromosomes. Careful tissue sampling techniques should theoretically provide more definitive results, but some physicians automatically assume that karyotype results showing a chromosomally normal female baby means that the tissue came from the mother and that the test is not conclusive. This can be frustrating for patients, because there is often no way to know whether the miscarried baby did have normal chromosomes, and to have a doctor tell you that there must have been an error with the tissue sample can feel dismissive.

What Role Do Chromosomal Anomalies Play in Miscarriage?

Cell division and chromosomes are complex subjects whose full biological explanation is beyond the scope of this book. In short, however, chromosomal anomalies occur when either the egg or the sperm had the wrong number of chromosomes or another chromosomal error at the time of fertilization. Cell division is such a complex process that it's very easy for something to go awry. This isn't something a person can influence, at least as far as modern medical science knows.

Exactly why some chromosomal anomalies result in miscarriage is another complex question. Some babies with an abnormal number of chromosomes can be born, as in the case of Down syndrome, which results from an extra copy of chromosome 21. But other chromosomal anomalies are "incompatible with life." At some point, the baby stops developing, because it lacks the genetic material to sustain life; the baby is subsequently miscarried.

Various studies have found differing percentages of miscarriage patients whose losses result from chromosomal anomalies. These differences probably derive from differences in the samples of people studied. The literature seems unclear on the exact role of chromosomal problems in repeated miscarriages. One study of couples who underwent preimplantation genetic diagnosis (genetic testing of eggs after in vitro fertilization) found that the majority of fertilized eggs tested had chromosomal abnormalities. Another study compared karyotypes from 122 repeat miscarriages to those from 133 first miscarriages. Only 25.4 percent of the karyotypes from repeat miscarriages were chromosomally abnormal, whereas 42.1 percent from the first miscarriages were abnormal. Further studies will most likely shed more light on the issue.

The risk of miscarriage due to chromosomal issues increases as parents, including fathers, age. Even in women older than 36, however, other conditions can cause recurrent miscarriages. No one who has had multiple losses should assume that the underlying reason is chromosomal unless a karyotype analysis indicates that it is.

What Causes the Anomalies in the First Place?

Imagine how much heartbreak could be saved around the world if we could figure out why cells won't divide correctly. Not only could practitioners prevent miscarriages, they could probably also slow the aging process.

While we don't know exactly what causes chromosomal anomalies, we know of a few factors that correlate with them. You don't necessarily have control over all these factors, and it would be impossible to prove that one of them caused a particular miscarriage. For each of the following factors, however, a body of evidence suggests a statistical relationship with increased rates of chromosomal anomalies in either the egg or the sperm.

* Hormonal disturbances

* Electromagnetic radiation (a controversial, less well-established factor)

* Exposure to petrochemicals

* Pollution

* Maternal or paternal smoking

* Alcohol consumption

* Random error in the cell-division process

* A maternal or paternal balanced translocation (see page 38)

* Maternal age

You're probably well aware of the dangers of smoking and drinking alcoholic beverages while trying to get (or remain) pregnant. You may not know, however, that petrochemicals, other chemical pollutants, and radiation are all suspected as causes of miscarriage. Environmental contaminants aren't always easy to avoid, in part because chemicals that haven't been proven beyond a doubt to cause miscarriage or other health problems are generally not well regulated. But it's wise to avoid exposure to radiation and chemicals known to be toxic both while you're trying to conceive and while you're pregnant.

The link between tap-water contaminants and miscarriage is controversial and not yet well understood. Many women prefer to play it safe by drinking bottled water before and after getting pregnant. Legal standards for bottled water, however, are generally the same as for municipal tap water. Before spending money on bottled water, you might consider having your household water tested, especially if it comes from a well. Test kits are available that can detect the most common toxins and let you know if there's cause for alarm, and commercial laboratories can do more complex tests.

Before you worry too much about environmental pollution (I know it's hard not to worry when you're desperate for a baby!), remember that, if other women in your neighborhood are getting pregnant and having healthy babies, there is little reason to believe that local pollution is preventing you from doing the same.

Remember, too, that chromosomal anomalies can originate in the sperm as well as the egg. When you are planning a pregnancy, your partner should take the same precautions that you take to avoid exposure to toxins.

Parental Translocations

During cell division, sometimes a piece of a chromosome will break off and attach to another chromosome. This can happen in a balanced or unbalanced manner. In a balanced translocation, the person who results has all the necessary genetic material, but some of it is stuck in an unusual place. For example, if a piece of chromosome 13 breaks off and gets stuck to chromosome 14, the person ends up with one normal chromosome 13 and one normal chromosome 14, and then a copy of chromosome 13 that is missing a piece and a copy of chromosome 14 that has the missing piece of chromosome 13 stuck to it.

A person does not necessarily have any negative health effects from a balanced translocation such as this. But when the person, man or woman, tries to have children, there is a 50 percent risk of miscarriage in each pregnancy. Why? Because when the cells divide, the sperm or egg gets only half the parent's chromosomes. In the case just described, the sperm or egg could end up with an *unbalanced* translocation—for example, a copy of chromosome 13 that is missing a piece and a copy of chromosome 14 that is normal. This would leave the fertilized egg with missing DNA. Or the sperm or egg could get too much genetic material—that is, a normal copy of chromosome 13 and a copy of chromosome 14 with an extra piece of chromosome 13 stuck to it. For a healthy pregnancy to occur, the sperm or egg cells need to divide either with the normal chromosomes or with both copies of the translocated chromosomes. This means the sperm or egg of a person with a balanced translocation has a 50 percent chance of having either both of the normal chromosomes or both of the translocated chromosomes, and a 50 percent chance of having missing or extra genetic material.

Another type of translocation is the robertsonian translocation. This type involves entire arms of chromosomes rather than smaller sections. The long arms of chromosome 21 could, for example, attach to the long arms of chromosome 15 to form a chromosome. Then the short arms could also join together, or they could be lost (in the chromosomes most commonly affected by robertsonian translocations, the short arms do not contain essential genetic material). In such cases, all the necessary genetic material is present, but when the cells divide to create sperm or egg cells there is a 50 percent chance that the resulting cells will have missing or extra genetic material.

What does this mean for you? Well, in 3 to 5 percent of couples who have recurrent miscarriages, at least one partner carries a balanced translocation. You and your partner might undergo karyotype analysis to find out if you're in this group. If you are, you might be advised to continue trying until you end up with a viable pregnancy, or you might be offered in vitro fertilization with preimplantation genetic diagnosis (that is, genetic testing of each fertilized egg). The latter approach has been shown to greatly reduce the miscarriage rate for parents who are carriers of balanced or robertsonian translocations, but even those couples who decide just to continue trying are likely to have a healthy infant eventually.

INFECTIONS

A few types of genital bacterial infections are associated with increased rates of miscarriage. These infections may cause a grayish or white vaginal discharge with a fishy odor, and sometimes itching or burning, but some women have no symptoms at all. Some physicians will test for infection when a woman has any abnormal vaginal discharge, but others will go straight to prescribing antibiotics, since the tests can be costly. Many practitioners are unaware that these infections can cause miscarriage, so you might consider printing one of the studies in the reference list before you ask about testing. If you have active symptoms that might indicate bacterial vaginosis, definitely ask your practitioner for a test before you try to conceive again.

ANATOMICAL PROBLEMS OF THE UTERUS

After chromosomal anomalies, the second most common cause of miscarriage is anatomical problems of the uterus. These problems are estimated to play a role in as many as 30 percent of repeat miscarriages. Uterine malformations occur in up to 4 percent of all women; other anatomical problems are much more common but less likely to cause miscarriages. The good news is that, in most cases, anatomical problems associated with miscarriage can be treated with surgery, and the woman can go on to carry a baby to term without complications.

Anatomical problems of the uterus at a glance

What are they? There are a number of uterine malformations that are congenital, such as septate uterus (see glossary), while other kinds, such as fibroids, occur in adulthood. Fibroids are growths in the uterus. Any of these conditions may prevent a pregnancy from developing properly. Cervical insufficiency, a condition in which the cervix dilates prematurely, is sometimes associated with uterine malformations.

Who is affected? Most of the time, uterine malformations are either hereditary or caused by environmental influences during the mother's prenatal development, such as exposure to a drug called DES, or diethylstilbestrol (see page 42).

Why do these problems cause miscarriage? Certain uterine shapes can make a woman more prone to having a weak cervix that cannot support a pregnancy, and other shapes may cause the egg to implant in a place where the uterus can't sufficiently nourish a pregnancy. Fibroids may interfere with implantation or nourishment of an implanted pregnancy.

What are the symptoms? Problems related to a weak cervix usually cause second-trimester miscarriage following normal prenatal development, but some anatomical problems, such as septate uterus, can cause first-trimester losses and missed miscarriages (see page 9). Fibroids may be asymptomatic or may cause pain in the lower abdomen.

How do I know if I have one of these problems? Diagnostic imaging tests, such as hysterosalpingogram (HSG), can provide clues, but the best way to know for sure is to have a hysteroscopy, an examination of the uterus with a camera. Ultrasound and magnetic resonance imaging (MRI) may also be used in diagnosing some anatomical problems.

What can I do about it? Some problems can be fixed surgically before conception. Others are treated with a cervical cerclage (see page 95) early in pregnancy to prevent preterm delivery. Fibroids may be treated by myomectomy (see page 45).

How certain is it that uterine abnormalities cause miscarriages? This is unclear. Some women with uterine abnormalities carry their babies to term with no problems. In other cases, the abnormalities seem to be clearly related to a history of miscarriages, and a woman can go on to have a successful pregnancy upon correction.

Anatomical problems of the uterus fall into the following categories:

* Septate uterus

* Other uterine malformations

* Cervical insufficiency ("incompetent cervix," "weak cervix")

- Fibroids

- Polyps

- Asherman's syndrome (intrauterine adhesions)

Septate uterus, or uterine septum, and other congenital uterine anomalies usually result from either heredity or exposure to a particular drug during the mother's prenatal development. If your practitioner has ever asked whether your mother took diethylstilbestrol (DES), a medication once prescribed to prevent miscarriages, this is because DES eventually was found to cause congenital uterine abnormalities that could lead to miscarriages in daughters of women who took the drug. (Because the use of DES was discontinued in the early 1970s, this drug is not likely to be a factor in miscarriages among women under age 35.)

> DES was used many years ago in the mistaken belief that it could prevent miscarriages. We know today that, in addition to increasing the risk of a very rare vaginal cancer in exposed women, DES has caused decreased fertility and increased risk of pregnancy loss. Diagnosis of the uterine abnormality associated with DES can be easily accomplished with a properly done hysterosalpingogram (see page 82).
> —BARRY JACOBS, M.D., F.A.C.O.G., TEXAS FERTILITY, P.A.

Septate Uterus

The most common congenital uterine abnormality is a septate uterus. This problem originates when, during prenatal development, a wall of tissue, or septum, forms between the two halves of the fetal uterus. Later, in adulthood, the septum often lacks an adequate blood supply to support a baby that implants on it. At some point in its development the baby stops growing.

The septum can be partial or complete, and the chance of pregnancy loss probably varies accordingly, but, in general, women with septate uteruses have an elevated risk of miscarriage. Surgical treatment seems to improve pregnancy outcomes; one study found that surgery to correct uterine septa improved rates of successful pregnancy from 4.4 percent to 87.5 percent. Surgical correction, or septoplasty, usually involves the woman going under anesthesia and the physician, aided by hysteroscopy, removing the septum. Like any surgical procedure, removal of a uterine septum carries risks of complications.

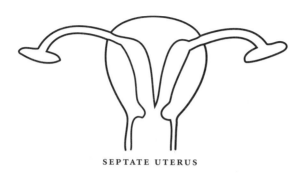

SEPTATE UTERUS

A fairly large proportion of women have some kind of uterine anomaly—maybe 1 to 5 percent of the population. . . . Plenty of women with uterine septa that we might never see have successful pregnancies.

—MARK P. LEONDIRES, M.D., F.A.C.O.G., MEDICAL DIRECTOR AND LEAD
PHYSICIAN, REPRODUCTIVE MEDICINE ASSOCIATES OF CONNECTICUT

Other Uterine Malformations

Although a septate uterus is the most common uterine malformation, others can increase the risk of miscarriage. According to one study, the unicornuate ("one-horned") uterus is the formation with the most reproductive complications. Didelphic ("double") and bicornuate ("two-horned") uteruses can also affect reproductive outcomes, including the risk of miscarriage. These uterine anomalies are important to address even when they are not linked to miscarriages, because they can also cause incompetent cervix (see page 44) and other problems that lead to extreme premature birth or stillbirth. This is why these structural abnormalities are among the first things that many physicians look for when evaluating a woman with recurrent miscarriages.

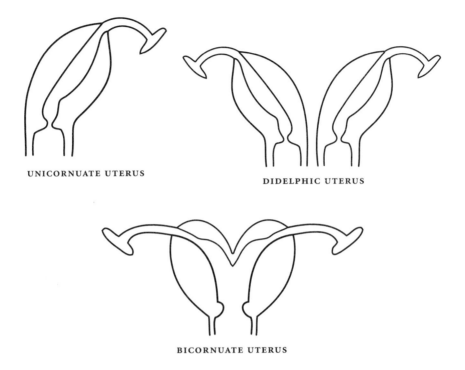

UNICORNUATE UTERUS

DIDELPHIC UTERUS

BICORNUATE UTERUS

Cervical Insufficiency

This is a new term that many practitioners are using for what used to be called "incompetent cervix" or "weak cervix," although you'll still hear the latter terms frequently. Cervical insufficiency is identified when, because of structural weakness or past injury, the cervix begins to dilate prematurely, with or without contractions. This can cause a baby to be born early—too early, in the most devastating cases, to survive outside the womb.

Cervical insufficiency can be associated with congenital uterine malformations, or it can result from trauma to the cervix, such as from repeated D&Cs. The cause is not always known. But about 25 percent of miscarriages that happen after 14 weeks (and probably a larger percentage of stillbirths and premature deliveries) are due to a weak cervix. If you have had a second-trimester loss, it is worth talking to your practitioner about whether you might have this condition. A common treatment is cervical cerclage, an operation to close the cervix with suture or surgical tape.

Fibroids

Fibroids are clusters of muscle cells and other tissue that grow in the wall of the uterus; some practitioners call them tumors. Fibroids come in different types and have widely varying impact on a woman's health and reproductive status. As many as 80 percent of all women may have some fibroids, according to the National Uterine Fibroids Foundation, but the fibroids cause problems in only about 25 percent of women who have them. No one knows what causes fibroids, but they may be genetic.

Most women with fibroids have no symptoms at all. After age 35, symptoms are more likely to occur. They can include pain in the uterine area, bleeding between periods, pain during sex, and feelings of fullness in the abdomen.

Even without symptoms, fibroids can cause infertility and pregnancy loss. Whether they do or not seems to depend on the location of the fibroids.

Fibroids can be diagnosed easily through an ultrasound exam, by imaging tests, or via laparoscopic exploratory surgery.

Treatment by myomectomy may improve pregnancy outcomes. Myomectomy is a surgery that involves removing the fibroids without taking healthy tissue from the uterus. There are other possible treatments for fibroids, but some (such as uterine artery embolization, a procedure that involves cutting off the blood supply to the fibroid, and the use of nonsteroidal anti-inflammatory drugs and hormones) have unknown effects on future pregnancies, and others (such as the use of birth control pills, which can reduce the pain and swelling of fibroids, and hysterectomy) would make pregnancy impossible. A woman who gets pregnant after a myomectomy may be advised to give birth by cesarean section.

Polyps

A polyp is an abnormal growth in a mucous membrane. Polyps in the uterus are common and usually not problematic, but some researchers suspect that they may increase miscarriage risks. Polyps can be surgically removed.

Asherman's Syndrome

This is a rare condition in which scar tissue has developed in the uterus, sometimes causing the sides of the uterus to stick together. Usually Asherman's syndrome develops after a D&C or other uterine surgery, but it can also result from a severe infection. Symptoms may include scant menstrual flow or none at all, although a woman with Asherman's syndrome who has no periods may feel pain at the time of the month when she would normally menstruate. The condition can both prevent conception and increase the risk of miscarriage. It can be treated with surgery.

How Do I Know if I Have an Anatomical Problem of the Uterus?

If you regularly experience pain with menstruation or during sex, you should certainly let your practitioner know, because this could indicate some type of uterine anomaly that could be linked to miscarriage. But even if you have no pain, a uterine abnormality is still a possibility. One study has indicated that it's prudent to run tests for uterine anomalies in women who have had two miscarriages rather than to wait for a third. A variety of different tests can be used to detect uterine anomalies, including hysterosalpingogram, hysteroscopy, laparoscopy, three-dimensional ultrasound, magnetic resonance imagery (MRI), and hysterosonography. Read more about these in chapter 3.

HORMONAL IMBALANCES

Hormonal problems are one of the most controversial possible causes of miscarriage, second only to immunological problems. Hormones are a complicated subject that few people understand well, save specialists in endocrinology. But a good body of research suggests that hormonal imbalances are correlated with miscarriages, and a few specific types of hormonal imbalances appear to cause miscarriages. So, without attempting more than a very basic explanation of how hormones function in the body, I'll try to address how they affect your miscarriage risk. If you are diagnosed with hormonal problems and want to know more, you might want to conduct further research.

These are a few hormonal conditions that may be related to miscarriage:

* Luteal-phase defect

* Polycystic ovarian syndrome

* Hyperprolactinemia

* Thyroid disease

The levels of reproductive hormones peak at different points during the menstrual cycle. The graph below illustrates when each hormone is at its highest level in an average 28-day cycle.

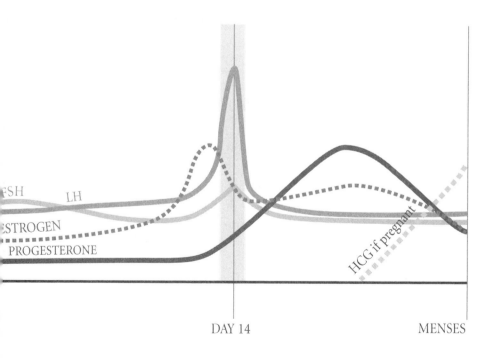

Hormonal imbalances at a glance

What are they? Abnormalities in a woman's hormones, such as progesterone, prolactin, follicle-stimulating hormone (FSH), or hormones produced by the thyroid.

Who is affected? Hormonal imbalances can have any number of causes. They can occur sporadically, or they can be chronic problems. There is no way to tell after the fact whether a hormonal problem caused a miscarriage.

How can they cause miscarriages? Elevated levels of some hormones may cause the eggs to be released before they are fully mature, and abnormal levels of others may affect the climate in the uterus so that it cannot support a pregnancy.

What are the symptoms? It's hard to tell who has hormonal problems and who doesn't, but a history of irregular menstrual cycles is a red flag. Hormonal imbalances can also cause weight gain or loss, acne, mood swings, premenstrual syndrome, and a variety of other symptoms. But even women without hormonal imbalances can experience these symptoms, so they are not definitive.

Luteal-phase Defect

If you've had more than one miscarriage, spent any time in an online miscarriage-support forum, or searched the Internet to learn about miscarriage, chances are you have already heard of progesterone. Progesterone is a hormone of the female reproductive system that increases during the final two weeks of the menstrual cycle, after ovulation. During this period, progesterone is produced by the corpus luteum ("yellow body"), which develops from the emptied ovarian follicle. If a woman becomes pregnant, the corpus luteum continues to produce progesterone, which maintains the uterine lining so that it can nourish a baby. Progesterone produced by the corpus luteum is thus key in sustaining a pregnancy in the first trimester. When the placenta matures, it takes over progesterone production.

How do I know if I have a hormonal imbalance? Blood tests are the best diagnostic tool for most hormonal problems, but some doctors will perform endometrial biopsy to diagnose one kind of hormonal condition, called luteal-phase defect (see page 48).

What can I do about it? Many practitioners believe that, after two or more consecutive miscarriages, women should be tested and treated for any hormonal abnormalities before attempting pregnancy again. Medications can help normalize hormone levels, as can certain lifestyle changes. Not all practitioners believe in treating hormonal imbalances with medication.

How certain is it hormonal imbalances cause miscarriages? The evidence is inconsistent. Women with recurrent miscarriages do tend to have hormonal imbalances, but therapies to correct the imbalances have not yet been proven effective in reducing miscarriage rates in double-blind, randomized trials. As a result, you'll find varying opinions in the medical community of the role of hormones in miscarriages. Many factors remain unknown.

Low progesterone in the second half of the menstrual cycle is usually called "luteal-phase deficiency" or "luteal-phase defect." Theoretically, an insufficient progesterone level could cause a first-trimester miscarriage, because the uterine lining would be unable to support the developing baby. Some practitioners believe that an insufficient uterine lining may cause miscarriage at around four to five weeks of gestational age. Others believe that low progesterone is a factor in infertility but not in miscarriages. Low progesterone may not cause miscarriage but may instead be associated with any pregnancy that fails. If a pregnancy is affected by chromosomal problems, for example, no amount of progesterone will help; administering progesterone supplements may postpone a miscarriage but will not prevent it.

The usual means of screening for luteal-phase defect is by checking a woman's progesterone level in a blood sample drawn at seven or eight days past ovulation (see page 79). The gold-standard test for diagnosing this defect is an endometrial biopsy to evaluate the uterine lining, although this is much more invasive than a blood test. Even with a biopsy, diagnosis may be difficult, because a woman can have a luteal-phase defect in one cycle but not the next, or the problem can be recurrent.

Not all practitioners are willing to treat for luteal-phase defect. Those who do may prescribe progesterone supplements (see page 87) or Clomid (see page 90).

Polycystic Ovarian Syndrome (PCOS)

This complex problem has been the subject of entire books. The National Women's Health Information Center estimates that 5 to 10 percent of women of childbearing age have the disorder, and among women known to have PCOS the miscarriage rate may be as high as 40 percent, although some handle pregnancy just fine. The cause of the disorder is not known, but women affected by it have a number of characteristic hormonal imbalances and characteristic cysts on the ovaries. The disorder also comes with a number of distressing symptoms, including systemic hormonal imbalances, a tendency toward obesity, unusual facial hair growth, acne, lack of a regular menstrual period, and more. Miscarriage rates in women with PCOS are elevated even among those who have undergone in vitro fertilization.

Researchers have studied several possible mechanisms that could explain why women with PCOS have a higher risk of miscarriage. At this writing, there are a number of competing theories about what the mechanism might be. The general consensus, however, is that something about the hormonal imbalances that women with PCOS suffer causes the eggs to be released before they are fully mature. One study suggests that the association of PCOS with miscarriages could occur because women with PCOS are prone to obesity, and obesity is an independent risk factor for miscarriage that comes along with hormonal problems. Other studies indicate that abnormally high or low levels of individual hormones, such as luteinizing hormone (which stimulates the ovaries to release the egg and plays a role in regulating the menstrual cycle), could be responsible. Other studies blame prolactin (see page 51), and still others blame insulin resistance, a prediabetic condition, which is associated with miscarriages even in women without PCOS or progesterone deficiencies.

If you have been diagnosed with PCOS or suspect you may have it, I highly recommend that you go over your options with a reproductive endocrinologist and refer to the relevant resources listed in Appendix B. A few treatments are showing great promise, primarily those involving the drug metformin and weight reduction (although I know firsthand that losing weight is much easier said than done). You'll find some discussion of these treatments in chapter 3.

Hyperprolactinemia

Prolactin, a hormone produced by the pituitary gland, stimulates development of the breasts during pregnancy in preparation for milk production and breastfeeding after a baby is born. Prolactin also suppresses progesterone production, which is part of the reason that women who are breastfeeding sometimes don't have menstrual cycles.

Excess prolactin is one of several hormonal imbalances that have been tied to increased miscarriage risk by multiple studies. The condition is referred to as hyperprolactinemia, and it is usually treated with a medication such as bromocriptine or cabergoline, which lower prolactin levels and have been shown to reduce the rate of miscarriages associated with the condition. A milky discharge from your nipples, if you are not currently breastfeeding, may be a sign of excess prolactin and should be mentioned to your physician.

The cause of elevated prolactin is unclear, but on rare occasions the elevation is associated with a tumor of the pituitary gland, so if you have high prolactin levels your practitioner may suggest that you undergo magnetic resonance imaging (MRI) to rule this out as a cause.

Thyroid Disease

Although it could be considered a maternal disease or an autoimmune problem, thyroid disease is classed with hormonal problems here because the condition manifests itself as elevated or reduced levels of thyroid hormones, such as free T4 (thyroxine) and TSH (thyroid-stimulating hormone). Like other hormonal problems that are related to miscarriage, thyroid disease would require many pages to discuss in depth. Following is a brief overview.

There are three common abnormal thyroid conditions: hypothyroidism (insufficient production of thyroid hormones), hyperthyroidism (excess production of thyroid hormones), and antithyroid antibodies. Hypothyroidism and hyperthyroidism are correlated with an increased risk of miscarriage. Hypothyroidism can increase the risk of miscarriage even in a subclinical case—one without obvious symptoms—so practitioners will commonly screen for hypothyroidism as a part of a miscarriage workup. Antithyroid antibodies have been suspected by some to be associated with miscarriage also; one study found a link, but more recent studies show that this condition probably does not increase the risk of miscarriage.

Early studies indicate that treating hypo- and hyperthyroid conditions with medications may improve pregnancy outcomes and reduce miscarriage rates.

BLOOD-CLOTTING DISORDERS

Women with a history of recurrent miscarriages are generally tested for (1) hereditary clotting factors and (2) MTHFR and homocysteine. More such factors may be discovered; research indicates that women who have recurrent miscarriages but test negative for these factors are at increased risk for episodes of deep vein thrombosis, or blood clots in the veins. This suggests that some clotting tendencies may be yet undiscovered.

Hereditary Clotting Factors

Specific gene mutations are thought to make carriers more likely to suffer from blood clots. These mutations include factor V Leiden, factor II, protein C deficiency, protein S deficiency, antithrombin deficiency, and factor II G20210A prothrombin. Some studies conclude they have a strong association with pregnancy problems and other studies find no such association at all.

We routinely check for factor V Leiden. If the mutation is present and is a homozygous mutation, we might want to treat the patient.

—PAOLO RINAUDO, M.D., PH.D., ASSISTANT PROFESSOR OF
REPRODUCTIVE ENDOCRINOLOGY AND INFERTILITY,
UNIVERSITY OF CALIFORNIA, SAN FRANCISCO

Blood-clotting disorders at a glance

What are they? Specific genetic abnormalities or antibodies that make your blood more likely than normal to form clots; these are also known as thrombophilias.

Who gets them? Many people carry thrombophilia gene mutations, but not everyone who carries blood-clotting factors will experience pregnancy loss.

Why do they cause miscarriages? This is not clear. It may be that blood clots interfere with the development of the placenta.

What are the symptoms? You can have a blood-clotting disorder and have no symptoms at all. Often, recurrent miscarriages are the first sign of the problem.

How do I know if I have this problem? Blood tests can check your clotting time or check for specific antibodies.

What can I do about it? Most clotting disorders are treated with heparin and low-dose aspirin.

How certain is it that this problem causes miscarriages? Many clotting factors are not well understood, and their link with miscarriage has not been conclusively proven.

A few studies indicate that women who have more than one factor predisposing them to thrombophilia are at the most risk for miscarriage. Women who are homozygous for (carry two copies of) a thrombophilia factor gene may also have a greater risk of miscarriage than women who are heterozygous (carry only one copy of the thrombophilia gene). What most practitioners do agree on is that more research is needed as to whether treating hereditary thrombophilias actually prevents miscarriages. In the meantime, you will find some practitioners testing for and treating hereditary thrombophilias and others holding back until more evidence surfaces.

MTHFR and Homocysteine

MTHFR (methylenetetrahydrofolate reductase) is still another factor that some practitioners test for and treat aggressively, while others laugh at the mere mention of it. Like the hereditary thrombophilias just discussed, MTHFR involves a gene mutation. It has two most commonly discussed forms, known as C677T and A1298C. As with most genes, you will have either one or two copies of the mutation. If you have one copy, the mutation is heterozygous; if you have two copies, the mutation is homozygous.

A few studies have associated MTHFR gene mutations with increased risk of miscarriages. But other studies have found no such association, at least when considering the mere presence of the gene and not its possible effects. Half the population have one copy of the MTHFR gene mutation, and 1 to 20 percent of the population have two copies, so the gene mutation itself probably isn't a root cause of miscarriages. But carriers of the gene are more likely than other women to have high levels of homocysteine, an amino acid that at high levels may lead to blood clots and other cardiovascular problems, and low levels of folate, or folic acid (see page 91). Both high homocysteine and low folate are independently related to higher-than-average rates of miscarriage.

Another theory is that the MTHFR gene plays a role in pregnancy loss because of interactions of the mother's genes with those of the unborn baby. Although some researchers hypothesize that MTHFR increases the risk of thrombophilia, it seems likely that any such link is related to the tendency of MTHFR to cause higher homocysteine levels and lower folate levels. For this reason, some practitioners believe that checking homocysteine levels in the blood is more sensible than testing for the MTHFR gene. Not everyone with the MTHFR gene tests high for homocysteine, but the risk of high homocysteine levels is greater among women with this gene. Treatment of MTHFR is generally considered unnecessary unless homocysteine levels are high.

The relationship between homocysteine levels and miscarriage is poorly understood, but high levels may cause improper development of blood vessels in the placenta. Nutritional supplementation with folic acid, vitamin B_6, and vitamin B_{12} has been shown to reduce homocysteine levels and so may reduce miscarriage risk, although this hasn't been proven. One controversial study has shown that heparin may also reduce homocysteine levels. A few practitioners prescribe heparin for women with MTHFR and elevated homocysteine, but others feel that the use of heparin is too aggressive unless the woman has had a blood clot.

Homocysteine is probably not a major factor in recurrent miscarriage. It may be one of the factors; the literature is not very clear on the outcome and benefits of treating high homocysteine levels. The association between MTHFR and recurrent miscarriages is not very clear, either. Some studies are controversial. It may be one of the factors, but I don't think it's going to be responsible by itself—not like factor V Leiden.

— PAOLO RINAUDO, M.D., PH.D.

A final note on thrombophilia: If you have been diagnosed with any thrombophilia, please be sure to discuss the matter with a general physician. Because thrombophilia may carry cardiovascular and other health risks, these conditions can affect not just your reproductive health but also your long-term overall health.

IMMUNOLOGICAL MALFUNCTIONS

The theory regarding immunological causes of miscarriage is that, in some women, something in the immune system goes awry and causes the mother's body to attack the unborn baby. These reactions can be *autoimmune,* which means the immune system reacts against one's own body, as with rheumatoid arthritis, or *alloimmune,* which means the reaction is against something foreign, such as a transplanted kidney. The mechanisms by which immune reactions may cause miscarriages are not well understood, and there is little evidence to support many of the treatments for these theoretical problems. Are the treatments useless, or are the wrong patients being selected for the studies? It is too soon to tell; the research is still ongoing.

Immunological malfunctions at a glance

What are they? Abnormalities in the mother's immune system. Antiphospholipid syndrome (APS) and antinuclear antibodies (ANAs) cause autoimmune reactions; human leukocyte antigen (HLA) system problems and natural killer cells cause alloimmune reactions.

Who is affected? Research results are inconclusive. Some immunological abnormalities are probably genetic, whereas others may be environmentally induced.

Why do they cause miscarriages? If current hypotheses are correct, the mother's immune system either forms antibodies against the baby or interferes with development of the placenta.

What are the symptoms? No symptoms would indicate this cause of miscarriage, except possibly an analysis of the placenta by a specialist in reproductive immunology.

How do I know if I have this problem? Blood tests can check your HLA genotype (see page 58) or level of natural killer cells (see page 60).

What can I do about it? Treatments include injecting the father's white blood cells into the mother, giving her prednisone, and using intravenous immunoglobulin (IVIg). The treatment for APS is generally heparin and low-dose aspirin.

How certain is it that this problem causes miscarriages? Heparin and low-dose aspirin are known to reduce the miscarriage rate in women with APS. Treatments for other immunological causes of recurrent miscarriage are highly controversial. The most widely accepted studies have found these treatments to be no more effective than placebos in reducing miscarriage rates, but practitioners who believe in the treatments assert that more research is needed.

These are the immunological factors that may be associated with recurrent miscarriage:

* Antiphospholipid syndrome

* Antinuclear antibodies

* Human leukocyte antigens

* Natural killer cells

As with hormonal and blood-clotting disorders, immunological disorders may have more than one of these factors, and they may be interrelated.

Antiphospholipid Syndrome (APS)

APS is an autoimmune condition in which a person has antibodies to certain fatty acids that occur naturally in the blood. Because a fairly solid body of scientific literature supports the relationship between APS and miscarriage, tests for antiphospholipid antibodies are a standard part of any miscarriage workup. The most common of the antibodies tested for are anticardiolipin and lupus anticoagulant (a positive result for lupus anticoagulant does not mean that you have or will develop the disorder called lupus, or systemic lupus erythematosus). Except in extremely severe cases, APS has no outward symptoms. Commonly, recurrent miscarriage is the first indication that a woman has this syndrome.

APS may cause miscarriages by various mechanisms. Antiphospholipid antibodies block the production of hCG from the placental cells; they block the growth and development of the placental cells; and they cause an inflammatory reaction.

APS is hard to diagnose. The medical community does not yet appear to have reached consensus on the diagnostic criteria; some sources indicate that certain antiphospholipid antibodies are more likely to be associated with miscarriage than others. In addition, the diagnostic tests seem to have limitations; a single positive test for an antiphospholipid antibody, or a single abnormal test of clotting time, may not be significant, and many practitioners diagnose APS only after a woman tests positive for certain antibodies more than once. The quality of the testing is important; the test sample should be sent to a reputable laboratory.

You may find some disagreement also over whether APS can be responsible for early as well as late miscarriages, although research indicates an association with both.

Injections of heparin, an anticoagulant drug, combined with low-dose aspirin have been shown to reduce the miscarriage rate in women with APS. Some practitioners recommend this treatment to all pregnant women who have at least one APS marker, but others recommend it only in severe cases, because low-dose aspirin and heparin may together cause pregnancy complications. When the medications are administered in the proper dosage, however, complications are rare.

A ny woman who has a thrombophilia, lupus anticoagulant, or antiphospholipid antibodies needs to make lifelong changes. These include (1) avoiding oral contraceptives, (2) taking 81 milligrams of aspirin per day, (3) avoiding tobacco use, (4) losing weight if she is overweight, and (5) correcting her cholesterol level as needed.

—WILLIAM H. KUTTEH, M.D., PH.D., H.C.L.D, DIRECTOR OF
FERTILITY ASSOCIATES OF MEMPHIS, MEMPHIS FERTILITY
LABORATORY, AND REPRODUCTIVE LABORATORY

Antinuclear Antibodies (ANAs)

Some research suggests that these antibodies, which attack the nucleus of the cell, may be linked to miscarriage. ANAs are most commonly associated with the disease systemic lupus erythematosus and other autoimmune disorders, but ANA levels can be elevated even in women without such a disease. These antibodies may play a role in attacking the developing baby, although the evidence seems somewhat thin.

Human Leukocyte Antigens

An antigen is any substance that causes a response by the immune system. All the cells in your body contain various types of proteins, and human leukocyte antigens (HLAs) are genes that encode the proteins in the outer membranes of your cells. Your immune system uses HLAs to recognize cells as being part of you or as foreign invaders. Although these proteins are native to your body and do not provoke such attacks by your own immune system, they may be interpreted as antigens if they are transplanted into someone else and so provoke an alloimmune (see page 55) reaction. This is why people who need organ transplants must have "matching" donors.

Some groups of HLAs are identified by added letters, such as HLA-B and HLA-C. You can develop antibodies against HLA components, and this mechanism causes the rejection of transplanted organs and may possibly cause some autoimmune diseases. A full explanation of the HLA system is beyond the scope of this book, but you can learn more by consulting any medical immunology text.

So what does HLA have to do with miscarriages? Well, some researchers have theorized that the same system that could cause rejection of transplanted organs (foreign tissue) could also be responsible for rejection of a developing baby, who carries HLA distinct from that of the mother. Some research has been done on the relationship between recurrent miscarriage and HLA, particularly with certain genetic variations involving HLA-G, an HLA that interacts with the fetal tissues. Some researchers have theorized that HLA-G protects the placenta from natural killer cells (see page 60) or protects the placenta from attack in other ways, but these functions are still not well understood. One meta-analysis found that HLA-DR1 was also associated with increased susceptibility to miscarriage. In addition, certain HLA genotypes may predispose a woman to form anticardiolipin antibodies (a type of antiphospholipid antibody) and thus to be susceptible to antiphospholipid syndrome (see page 57). Some HLA genotypes may also predispose women with uterine anomalies to miscarry. Another theory that ties the HLA system to miscarriages is this: When parents share similarities in their HLA genotypes, the mother's body may not recognize the differences, and so may fail to develop "blocking antibodies" to stop her immune system from attacking the fetus. Proposed treatments include injections of the father's white blood cells into the mother to boost this immune recognition, and to give the mother infusions of intravenous immunoglobulin (IVIg).

Even if HLA variations are statistically correlated with higher rates of miscarriage, the treatments are unproven. Meta-analysis has revealed no proof that these treatments are any more effective than placebos, although critics assert that existing studies have not screened patients properly and that better screening criteria should be developed. Anyone considering treatment for HLA problems should be aware that the treatment may or may not work; it's just too early to tell.

Natural Killer Cells

These are normal white blood cells that serve key functions within the immune system. Elevated levels of natural killer cells have been found in patients who experience recurrent miscarriage, and some researchers (but not all) believe this may reflect the attack of the mother's overactive immune system against the fetus. Abnormalities in the level of natural killer cells may also be tied to the HLA-G genotype abnormalities already discussed. A few studies suggest that a woman's level of natural killer cells may predict her miscarriage risk even before conception, although this research is still preliminary. Treatments for elevated natural killer cells are similar to those used for HLA genotype abnormalities, but these

Author's Story

I was curious about immunological treatments when I went to my first appointment with a reproductive endocrinologist following my third miscarriage. I had a family history of autoimmune disorders, and I wondered if something related could be at work in my miscarriages. But the doctor warned me that evidence had not yet proven the efficacy of immunological treatments for miscarriage, and he felt they had no place in medicine outside of clearly identified clinical trials. He added that he felt many of the people promising immunological treatments as miracle cures for recurrent miscarriage were doing so to make money off desperate people. I don't know how true all that is, but, after researching these treatments, I think it wise to use caution before proceeding with them. They may yet prove useful, but I'd first try everything else that has more established evidence of efficacy. Even if these methods work, probably only a small minority of miscarriage patients actually need them. If you pursue them anyway, look for a clinic with a lot of expertise and a proven track record.

treatments have not been proven effective compared to placebos. They may eventually be shown to work for some carefully screened patients, but it's just too early to say.

MATERNAL ILLNESS

If you have one of the chronic diseases that are linked to recurrent miscarriage, you probably knew you had it before you started trying to get pregnant, you are most likely working closely with a medical professional to manage your disease, and your practitioner has probably already explained the risks that your disease carries in pregnancy. This section is therefore just a brief overview of why these diseases are linked to miscarriage.

These are the conditions currently linked to miscarriage risk in pregnancy:

* Cancer

* Diabetes

* Systemic lupus erythematosus

* Uncontrolled hypertension

* Kidney disease

* Obesity and anorexia

* Celiac disease

Cancer

Chemotherapy during the first trimester may increase the risk of miscarriage, and studies disagree about its safety during the second and third trimesters. Treatment with radioactive agents in the year prior to a pregnancy can also increase miscarriage rates. Some literature suggests that having had radiation therapy to the abdominal area in particular increases the risk of pregnancy complications, including miscarriage, for cancer survivors. All of these increased risks are probably due to increases in the rate of chromosomal abnormalities. Someone with cancer who is actively undergoing chemotherapy should not purposely get pregnant,

Maternal illness at a glance

What is it? A disease in the mother that carries an increased risk of miscarriage.

Who is at risk? Most of these diseases are genetic or have unknown causes.

Why do these diseases cause miscarriage? This varies by disease; some place too much stress on the woman's body or interfere with development of the placenta.

What are the symptoms? This varies by disease; some, such as subclinical celiac disease, may have no obvious symptoms.

How do I know if I have one of these diseases? If you suspect you have any of these illnesses, discuss the matter with your doctor.

What can I do about it? The treatment varies by disease.

How certain is it that this problem causes miscarriages? Although many of these diseases are associated with higher-than-average rates of miscarriage, the reason is not always known.

and if you've been diagnosed with cancer in the past, checking with your practitioner before trying to conceive will give you the best odds.

Diabetes

Poorly controlled diabetes of both types, 1 and 2, is associated with an increased rate of miscarriage. When the disease is well controlled, however, the miscarriage risk is no higher than in women without diabetes. If you have diabetes, your best route to a good outcome is conceiving when you are at your healthiest and seeking subsequent monitoring by a high-risk pregnancy specialist.

Systemic Lupus Erythematosus (SLE)

Women with SLE, or lupus, were once counseled not to get pregnant at all, but these days such advice is rare. Women with lupus have a higher risk of miscarriage because of increased incidence of antiphospholipid antibodies (see page 57), so be sure to ask your doctor about a screening for these antibodies. Generally, as with other diseases, the best outcomes can be achieved by conceiving when the disease is well controlled. According to the Lupus Foundation of America, women who conceive after five to six months of remission of symptoms are less likely to experience a flare during pregnancy.

Women with SLE should consult with a physician to develop a plan before trying to conceive, to be sure that their current medication regime is okay during pregnancy, and to get some baseline tests, one of which may be a 24-hour total urine protein (a test in which the patient collects urine for 24 hours and then the protein is measured to evaluate kidney function). Women with lupus have an increased miscarriage rate and often deliver prematurely, sometimes due to blood-pressure elevation or poor fetal growth; however, many pregnancies will also go well. But a high level of obstetrical care is involved.
—Patricia Robertson, M.D., professor of clinical obstetrics and gynecology and specialist in maternal-fetal medicine at the University of California, San Francisco

Uncontrolled Hypertension

Only thin evidence associates hypertension, or high blood pressure, with recurrent miscarriage, but I discuss it here because a physician or two mentioned hypertension during my own struggle with miscarriages. The theory is that uncontrolled hypertension can interfere with the development of the placenta, and at least one study has suggested this, although the sample size was quite small. Hypertension later in pregnancy is associated with adverse outcomes as well, so, if you have high blood pressure before you get pregnant, try to get it under control prior to conception.

If you are taking medication for hypertension, be sure to consult with your doctor about whether your medication is safe for a developing baby. Your medication should not be in the category of ACE inhibitors.

Kidney Disease

It used to be that patients with kidney disease, like those with lupus, were advised not to get pregnant. Today, however, doctors know better how to manage pregnancy in women with kidney disease. Even women who have had kidney transplants are now able to have a fairly normal pregnancy. In women whose kidneys are failing, the risk of miscarriage is increased, probably because of the stresses that the disease and treatment place on the body. Clearly, you should not try to get pregnant if your kidneys are failing. If you have any kind of renal disease, in fact, you should consult with your physician to determine whether or not attempting pregnancy is a good idea, and work with a high-risk specialist if you do get pregnant. In milder kidney diseases, the biggest pregnancy risks are preeclampsia and gestational hypertension, not miscarriage.

Obesity and Anorexia

Obesity has been shown to be a risk factor for miscarriage, and it appears to be independent of factors such as polycystic ovarian syndrome and diabetes, although the reasons are not well understood at this point.

Anorexia also can increase the risk of miscarriage, probably by altering the body's metabolism. Some women with anorexia don't menstruate, and therefore can't get pregnant in the first place.

Both anorexia and obesity involve more than lifestyle choices and can have complex psychological or physiological roots. Neither condition is easily remedied. In either case, however, working toward a healthy body weight can reduce pregnancy risks. If you are overweight, please do not blame yourself for miscarrying. But taking steps to reduce your body weight may bring your hormones into a balance that could better support pregnancy. If you have polycystic ovarian syndrome (see page 50), your hormonal problems are probably causing a tendency toward being overweight.

If you decide to try to lose or gain weight, consider seeing a dietitian or nutritionist who can help you plan a diet that will benefit your overall health. Any kind of crash diet would only achieve short-term weight loss at the expense of your health.

Celiac Disease

This complex disorder involves intolerance to gluten, a protein found in wheat and several other cereal grains. The classic symptoms are gastrointestinal complaints, such as diarrhea and gas after eating foods containing gluten. The medical community once believed that celiac disease was rare, but new estimates indicate that as many as 1 in 133 people may have the disease. Many of these people may not exhibit any symptoms of the disease, however, and be unaware they have it.

Subclinical, or undiagnosed, celiac disease has recently been tied to miscarriage, although the research is still preliminary. Because celiac disease (and other undetected food intolerances) can damage the intestinal lining and the natural bacterial balance of the gut, affected individuals may have difficulty in absorbing key nutrients from foods or vitamin supplements, despite having a normal weight. It's possible that these undetected nutritional deficiencies are responsible for the increased risk of miscarriage. The treatment of celiac disease is typically to adopt a completely gluten-free diet, but the research has not yet shown whether a gluten-free diet reduces the miscarriage rate among women with the disorder.

LIFESTYLE FACTORS

Again, I am going to keep this section short, because if you are trying to have a baby you probably already know that you need to maintain a healthy lifestyle. But these are a few of the lifestyle factors that are or may be related to miscarriage:

* Smoking

* Use of street drugs

* Caffeine intake

Smoking

Women who smoke cigarettes may be as much as 80 percent more likely to miscarry than women who don't. Even heavy smoking by the father may increase the risk of miscarriage, possibly by increasing the risk of damage to the chromosomes in the sperm. A mother's exposure to secondhand

> ## Lifestyle factors at a glance
>
> *What are they?* Smoking, using street drugs, and consuming large quantities of coffee or other substances containing caffeine.
>
> *Why do they cause miscarriages?* Chemicals may pass to the developing baby and interfere with development of the placenta.
>
> *What can I do about this?* Give up potentially dangerous habits; get support if needed.
>
> *How certain is it that this problem causes miscarriages?* The evidence is conflicting, and the link between caffeine and miscarriages is especially controversial. But tobacco and some street drugs have widely accepted, strong causal links to miscarriage.

smoke may increase the risk of miscarriage, too, although studies have given conflicting answers to this question. Avoiding cigarette smoke is a wise move by anyone planning a pregnancy.

Use of Street Drugs

Drugs such as cocaine and methamphetamines are not good for anyone, not to mention pregnant women. Not all street drugs have been evaluated for links to miscarriage, but most are associated with negative pregnancy outcomes, including premature birth and health problems for the baby. All of these drugs should be avoided when trying to conceive and during pregnancy.

Caffeine Intake

The consumption of caffeine has been shown to correlate with miscarriages in multiple studies, most of which have shown an increased risk of miscarriage when the mother consumes five or more cups of coffee per day. Whether or not caffeine actually causes miscarriage is still being debated; the correlation may have other causes. For example, nausea in pregnancy is associated with good outcomes, and some researchers believe that women who have normal pregnancies are less likely to drink coffee, because the smell and taste make them nauseous. Few of the existing studies have accounted for such confounding factors, although one study has suggested that caffeine intake is a risk factor independent of nausea. It's also possible that certain genetic differences may make caffeine consumption risky for some women but not for others. For now, it is prudent to minimize caffeine intake if you are concerned about miscarriage. A common recommendation is to keep coffee intake to less than three cups a day.

STRESS

Let's say you are being chased by a tiger. The normal response is either to run or to try to hit the beast. This is called the fight-or-flight response. The body instantly produces a cascade of chemicals (such as adrenaline and cortisol) to get the body into maximum "save my life" mode.

The body responds exactly the same way whether the tiger is real or perceived. This means that any extreme stress (job loss, divorce, death of a loved one, diagnosis of infertility, miscarriage, etc.) triggers the exact same bodily response. The body does not produce "tiger adrenaline" or "I have just had a miscarriage adrenaline"; it just produces adrenaline.

In its best effort to allocate limited resources, the body shuts down nonessential parts. The last thing the body needs to do is conceive and reproduce when its life is in imminent danger from an attacking tiger.

Unless this fight-or-flight mechanism is switched off, a woman under stress is going to face a considerable hurdle in being able to conceive or carry to term.

—GERALD WILLIAMS, L.AC. (CALIFORNIA),
D.A. (RHODE ISLAND), M.S.T.O.M., CLINICAL DIRECTOR
AND FOUNDER, REPRODUCTIVE WELLNESS

More and more studies are showing that stress, especially the chronic kind, may be related to miscarriage. Experts who say it's a myth that stress causes miscarriage probably fear that women whose lives have been stressful will blame themselves for their pregnancy losses. If we have failed to control the amount of stress in our lives, or our reactions to stress, isn't this our own fault? But the news of a connection between stress and pregnancy loss can bring not only a vague feeling of guilt but also both hope and direction. If stress indeed causes miscarriage, it's important that we know this, so that we will do everything in our power to minimize our stress.

Let's look at the research. Cortisol is a hormone that your body produces when under stress, and a 2006 study showed that women with higher cortisol levels were more likely to have miscarriages. Other studies have found links between stress and immune-system or hormonal abnormalities that are linked independently to miscarriage. A few studies have found no link between stress and miscarriage. Some have suggested that the link can be explained by the increased tendency toward alcohol and drug abuse by women who are under stress (most studies have not controlled for alcohol and drug abuse).

Modern lives are very stressful. In days past, we'd be sitting around on a farm, and we'd go to bed early because we had no lights. And different people experience different effects from stress. We know that some women under stress stop having regular periods. This is an extreme example. Women under stress can also have an inadequate luteal phase, which doesn't lead to good support for early pregnancy. Reducing stress is every person's own project and responsibility.

—MARK P. LEONDIRES, M.D., F.A.C.O.G.

As with most other possible causes of miscarriage, the true risk of stress is unknown, but it may well be a causal factor in some cases. If this possibility is new to you, please do not succumb to the temptation to analyze your own loss and conclude that stress must have been the cause. Remember that if stress always caused miscarriages the human race would have ceased to exist long ago, because all pregnant women worry about their babies. Instead of focusing on the past, if you feel you are suffering from chronic stress right now, focus on trying to find ways to reduce it, because it's healthy to get rid of excess stress whether or not it may have caused you to miscarry. Use the possible link between stress and miscarriage as a motivator to take care of yourself.

Unknown Causes of Miscarriage

You can't always find a cause for a particular miscarriage. As stated earlier in this chapter, comprehensive recurrent miscarriage workups find a possible cause about 60 percent of the time. In other cases, the test results all come back normal, and women are left with no clue to what's preventing them from carrying a pregnancy to term.

If you're in this situation, you need to find a way to make peace with it. I know that this is much easier said than done. If you have seen a specialist, had all the pertinent tests run, and found nothing fixable, then you have two options. You can find a practitioner who's willing to try some experimental treatments just to see if they might work. Such practitioners are out there; many believe that progesterone or, less commonly, heparin may benefit the majority of recurrent miscarriage patients even in the absence of an identifiable cause. Ask nearly any physician who uses progesterone for this purpose, and you'll hear anecdotal evidence about its power, although this power isn't scientifically proven. Some physicians believe that patients whose losses have unknown causes may benefit from heparin anyway (see page 86). But when there isn't any clearly identifiable problem, only you and your practitioner can decide on the right course.

You can instead consider alternative treatments. Chapter 4 discusses various alternative treatments and therapies that may reduce stress or lower miscarriage risks. Most alternative therapies carry little risk, although some herbs should be used with caution, since a few may actually cause miscarriages. Although conventional tests may not have confirmed their usefulness, alternative therapies aren't necessarily useless.

Remember that your chances of ultimately achieving a healthy pregnancy remain high. One oft-cited study examined couples with recurrent miscarriages for which no cause could be found, and during the course of the study 75 percent of the women who conceived succeeded in carry-ing their babies to term. (The regular ultrasound scans and checkups provided to women in this study may have contributed to their high suc-cess rate by reducing their anxiety. See "Supportive Care," page 96.)

> *After the first miscarriage I was too scared to try again for six months. After the second I wanted to get pregnant as soon as possible to prove I could do it. For the next 19 months, getting pregnant became an obsession. We spent so much money on tests and weird treatments to improve our chances. After the third miscarriage I decided never to try again, and my husband was waiting to be sterilized when I miraculously got pregnant by accident.*
>
> —CASEY

CHAPTER 3

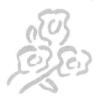

Miscarriage Testing and Treatments

MISCARRIAGES HAVE MANY POTENTIAL CAUSES and many unknowns. Even in antiphospholipid syndrome (see page 57), which seems to be most widely acknowledged as a definite cause of some miscarriages, there is disagreement over diagnostic criteria. In most losses, particularly early ones, the only time doctors can truly pinpoint a cause is when a karyotype (see page 34) shows chromosomal anomalies.

But once you've considered all the factors that might have caused your miscarriage, the obvious next question is what you can do to prevent another. I'll discuss that question in this chapter, starting with knowing when to seek help, then continuing to the tests you should expect or ask about, and ending with a look at a myriad of conventional treatments. I'll briefly discuss treatments that are still deemed experimental, which means they have a theoretical basis but remain unproven.

Remember that this chapter is not intended as medical advice but merely as a description of the options available and the rationale behind them. Address questions about these options to your chosen medical practitioner.

If You've Had One Miscarriage

Like the previous chapter, this one is most pertinent if you have had more than one miscarriage and have sought a workup for recurrent miscarriage. If you are reading this chapter after having had one loss, please keep it in perspective. In all likelihood, you will not need to worry about high-tech treatment. You probably do not have an underlying medical problem that caused your loss; the odds are high that your baby had a chromosomal anomaly, as described in chapter 2 (see page 33). I know this won't stop you from worrying, though, so I'd like to suggest you read the discussion in chapter 4 on stress relief and alternative treatments to boost fertility, and save this chapter to read later, if you need to. If you continue to worry and to wonder about a possible underlying cause for your loss, you might look for a practitioner who will agree to run at least a minimal workup.

Be aware, though, that testing for the causes of recurrent miscarriage can cost thousands of dollars, and many insurance companies will pay for these tests only after a couple have had three consecutive losses. If you have had just one miscarriage, you will almost certainly have to pay the costs yourself.

I was told I would have to miscarry again before any tests would be done. If you ask me, that is cruel! Why should I have to face another loss when testing could prevent future heartache?

—KIMBERLY

I was desperate to get pregnant after the first loss. After the second, I expected another. I wanted to get pregnant again just to get the miscarriage over with, because medical help was not available until you had had three miscarriages in a row. My partner felt the same.

—ROBIN

I cannot even think about trying to get pregnant again and risking another child's life without knowing what happened to the first.

—AMY

If You've Had More Than One Miscarriage

You may be frustrated with all the people who told you everything would be fine the second time you got pregnant. You may have celebrated your second pregnancy only to find yourself even more crushed than the first time you miscarried, because you allowed yourself to believe things were going to be okay. For you, seeing a positive pregnancy test probably brings feelings of anxiety and worry rather than joy and anticipation. You have lost your innocence about pregnancy, and you may be looking for anything that might help you understand what has happened to you and find a way to stop further losses. You may be so desperate for answers that you find it cathartic to read medical journals with the latest studies and findings on miscarriage.

In your search for information, you'll see statistics indicating that your chances of a successful pregnancy, even without treatment, are always higher than your odds of miscarrying. But don't let this stop you from seeking testing; many of the studies from which such statistics derive have excluded women with known conditions that may cause miscarriage.

With testing currently available, a potential miscarriage cause can be identified in about 60 percent of women with recurrent miscarriage. So if you're going to have tests done, either you'll identify a cause and treat it, and wait hopefully for your next pregnancy, or you won't find anything but can try again knowing that you've done everything you could to rule out an underlying cause and that odds remain high you'll eventually have a baby.

If you have had just two consecutive miscarriages, check with your insurance company before assuming the tests will be covered. Even if you have had three miscarriages, you may get a negative answer at first. Make sure the company representative understands that you are asking about recurrent miscarriage—a complication of pregnancy—and not infertility testing. You may have to point out that you conceived on your own, without treatment, and refer to the company's own statement of benefits. If your plan covers pregnancy and delivery, then it must also cover tests and treatment for recurrent miscarriage, at least after three losses if not after two.

In our clinic, we have spent 15 years or more writing articles, providing scientific information, and educating not only physicians but also insurance companies that the frequency of abnormal finding is the same in couples with two consecutive losses or with three. We are glad to report that many insurance companies now will cover an evaluation after two losses, although not all will.

— WILLIAM H. KUTTEH M.D., PH.D., H.C.L.D.

A Note on Scientific Proof

Most of the treatments described in this chapter are not widely accepted within the medical community, even though many are commonly used. Available scientific evidence regarding their efficacy is conflicting; some studies show certain treatments to be greatly beneficial, while others proclaim them useless. Some practitioners will offer every tool in the box to treat recurrent miscarriage, regardless of whether scientific consensus supports any of the treatments. Other practitioners refuse to treat miscarriages at all, because they feel that the treatments need more research before being used in clinical practice.

If you think about it, you can probably see the merits of both viewpoints. The first group of practitioners believes in using any treatment that may help, as long as it isn't likely to cause harm. But read a little bit about the debacle of the 1960s and 1970s involving DES (see page 42), and you'll understand how well-intentioned medicine can sometimes cause harm. Practitioners in the second group will often cite studies showing that a great majority of patients suffering recurrent miscarriage ultimately have healthy pregnancies even in the absence of treatment.

For many women, unfortunately, the second approach just doesn't cut it. For starters, many noninterventionists forget that the studies showing high success rates in the absence of treatment considered only idiopathic recurrent miscarriage cases, which means that before the study started the researchers screened out women whose miscarriages had obvious causes. This is important, because many who take the nonintervention stance dissuade women from having miscarriage workups. The success rates of patients with idiopathic recurrent miscarriage should be reassuring to anyone who has completed a miscarriage workup and found nothing to treat, but these statistics should not be quoted to women in place of testing to rule out known miscarriage causes.

For a large number of miscarriage patients, doing something that might help and probably won't hurt feels better than crossing one's fingers and doing nothing. Many women are willing to inject themselves with heparin just in case this might prevent another loss, even though if the pregnancy continues and a baby is born there is no way to know whether this would have happened in the absence of the treatment. Many women view themselves in each pregnancy as carrying an actual baby, not just a theoretical one. To them, the notion that one should just keep making more babies and waiting to see if they live or not, without even checking whether it is possible to improve their odds of survival, is absurd and insulting. With each pregnancy, for many women, the stakes are huge. It's not always easy to just "wait and see," and, if things go wrong, shrug one's shoulders and try again, hoping for better luck next time.

The "wait and see" approach has merit, too, however. It's true that most miscarriage treatments have not been adequately studied. For many of these treatments, research results are conflicting, and evidence of efficacy is lacking. And you never know which treatment could turn out to be the next DES, even though today's interventions are better monitored and appear to be safe. The caution many physicians exercise as they avoid jumping at every new "cure" without adequate data is part of the reason why we probably won't see another DES scandal.

The point is that there is no right approach to the treatment of recurrent miscarriage. You can tread cautiously by choosing only treatments that have withstood the most rigorous safety studies and have proven effective for specific problems that you know you have, and you can trust that the odds of having a baby rather than a miscarriage are always on your side. Or you can seek out anything and everything that might prevent miscarriage, and trust in the evidence that most of these treatments probably won't hurt even if they don't help. Or you can take a path somewhere in the middle.

When to Seek Testing

If you've miscarried once, the conventional wisdom is that you should try again, and seek testing only if you miscarry again. For most people, this is probably the best approach. Miscarriages most commonly *are* single incidents, and most women do go on to have a healthy pregnancy the next time. Yet testing after a first miscarriage may be worth consideration for some. For example, if you have miscarried in the second trimester, you may want to seek chromosomal testing, testing for blood-clotting factors, or an investigation of whether you have a uterine anomaly that causes cervical insufficiency (see page 44). If a treatable cause is identified, you may find some peace of mind in knowing what caused the loss and that it wasn't your fault, and you may be able to start your next pregnancy with a treatment plan.

The test for antiphospholipid syndrome is neither difficult nor terribly expensive, and this syndrome is one of few proven miscarriage causes with a treatment of well-documented efficacy. If you have an understanding practitioner, you might consider asking for this test after your first loss.

If you've had two miscarriages, there may be no reason to wait before seeking testing. Some doctors insist on waiting for the third miscarriage; they say that a woman who has had two miscarriages is only slightly more likely to miscarry in her next pregnancy than is someone who has had no miscarriages at all. A doctor is especially likely to say this if the patient's insurance company has a rule against paying for miscarriage testing before a third loss has occurred. Yet the American College of Obstetricians and Gynecologists found in February 2001 that the frequency of abnormal findings was the same in couples who had had two losses as in those who had had three. For your peace of mind, then, you should get the testing if you want it and if your insurance company will pay for it or you can afford to pay for it yourself. If your practitioner won't cooperate, consider finding a new one. More and more physicians support testing for possible causes after the second rather than the third miscarriage, to save unnecessary heartbreak for women who have treatable problems.

The likelihood of finding a cause for miscarriage goes down as women age. But anyone who has had two consecutive miscarriages, or three miscarriages with an intervening pregnancy, should have an evaluation and a workup.

—Mark P. Leondires, M.D., F.A.C.O.G.

Choosing the Right Practitioner

Most likely, your miscarriages were diagnosed by a family practitioner or obstetrician-gynecologist (OB-GYN). If you trust this practitioner and feel he or she has a good grasp of miscarriage research and treatments, then this practitioner may be a good one to see for your testing. Bear in mind, however, that most OB-GYNs and family practitioners do not spend the bulk of their time dealing with miscarriages. The average OB-GYN is more experienced with healthy pregnancies than with problems related to miscarriage, and he or she may not be up to speed on the latest research. Besides, you probably don't want to sit in a waiting room full of visibly pregnant women—a definite possibility in a general OB-GYN office—when you come into the office to discuss your miscarriages.

For these reasons, it might be best to seek a miscarriage specialist. In most cases, these are practitioners who also treat couples who have been unable to conceive. Specifically, you may want to seek a reproductive endocrinologist (RE). REs are OB-GYNs who have special training in managing the hormonal part of the reproductive system. Although these doctors can treat a range of hormonal problems, infertility and recurrent miscarriage are a large focus of many RE practices. You can find an RE or other fertility specialist with the resources in Appendix B.

Some OB-GYNs who lack RE certification also practice as fertility specialists. You might find such a doctor by asking around for referrals or by checking the Yellow Pages for OB-GYNs who mention infertility in their ads.

Your first appointment will likely include a review of your medical history. To expedite the evaluation, get your records from any other physicians you have seen and bring them with you to your appointment. Your records should include any blood tests, ultrasound scans, and genetic tests you have had. Your specialist will want to know when each test was done and whether you were pregnant at the time. Also bring along notes on what you remember of each pregnancy: when you got pregnant, your first symptoms of a miscarriage, when these symptoms occurred, and any other facts that may be relevant. All of this information will help the specialist determine what further tests are most appropriate for your circumstances.

Many patients call their doctor the day before their visit to a specialist, or even the day of the visit, and are surprised that their records have not miraculously shown up at the specialist's office. The patient needs to understand that pulling records is time-consuming, and that she should be responsible for picking up the records and carrying them to the specialist's office.
—WILLIAM H. KUTTEH, M.D., PH.D., H.C.L.D.

Remember that doctors work for you; *it's not the other way around. Be firm about what testing you want done.*

—NANCY

Ask a lot of questions of your doctor. No question is silly, stupid, or unnecessary. If you're confused, ask for clarification. Don't take everything the doctor says for granted. Doctors are human, too. Get another opinion if something doesn't seem right.

—SHERRY

Get all the testing you can. Read everything you can find. Soak up information like a sponge. Make a plan and get going.

—PAULA

Testing

Regardless of which practitioner you choose to see, wading through the many possible tests can be overwhelming. Figure 3.1 on page 81 illustrates the typical selection of available tests in a miscarriage workup. I hope your practitioner will make him- or herself available to explain whether or not you need these tests and what they mean, but in general, this is what you may be facing.

This book will not discuss what results are normal or abnormal for any specific test. I cannot interpret test results because I am not a physician, and because what is normal for one person may be abnormal for the next. In addition, normal values may vary by lab.

Figure 3.1 is a graphic representation of some testing and treatment options for recurrent pregnancy loss.

BLOOD TESTS

The majority of miscarriage tests are blood tests, and most of these blood tests measure hormonal levels or identify blood-clotting factors. The following lists provide the names of specific tests and their purposes.

Tests for Hormone Levels

* Day 2–3 FSH and LH: Checks for abnormalities with follicle-stimulating hormone (see page 187) and luteinizing hormone (see page 188) on the second or third day of the menstrual cycle, or a day or two after your period starts.

* Day 21 progesterone: Checks for luteal-phase deficiency (see page 48). Although this test is usually given on day 21 of the menstrual cycle, the test should actually be done seven days past ovulation. If you do not have 28-day cycles, you should alert your practitioner of this. You may need to take the test on a different day.

* Prolactin: Checks for abnormal elevation. Many practitioners test for prolactin (see page 51) at the same time as progesterone.

- Androgen panel: Looks for hormonal elevations characteristic of polycystic ovarian syndrome (see page 50). The hormones tested for are usually testosterone and DHEAS (dehydroepiandrosterone sulfate).

- Thyroid panel: Checks for abnormalities of thyroid hormones, which could indicate thyroid disease or malfunction.

Tests for Blood-clotting Factors

- Anticardiolipin antibodies and lupus anticoagulant: This test checks for signs of antiphospholipid clotting abnormalities (see page 57).

- aPTT (activated Partial Thromboplastin Time): This test checks for abnormalities in blood-clotting times.

- ANA (antinuclear antibody): These antibodies may indicate immune system problems.

- APC (activated protein C): This protein may be associated with hereditary thrombophilia (see page 53), which may be linked to miscarriage.

- Protein S, protein C, or antithrombin III deficiency: The lack of these factors may also be linked with hereditary thrombophilia.

- FVL (factor V Leiden): This gene mutation is also associated with hereditary thrombophilia.

- Prothrombin II gene: This gene is another hereditary cause of thrombophilia.

Other Blood Tests

- Parental karyotypes: Checks for a balanced translocation or another chromosomal anomaly that would cause miscarriage (see page 38).

- MTHFR: Many practitioners will test for this gene mutation, even though the value of the test is disputed (see page 54).

Figure 3.1: Tests, Diagnoses, and Treatments for Recurrent Miscarriage

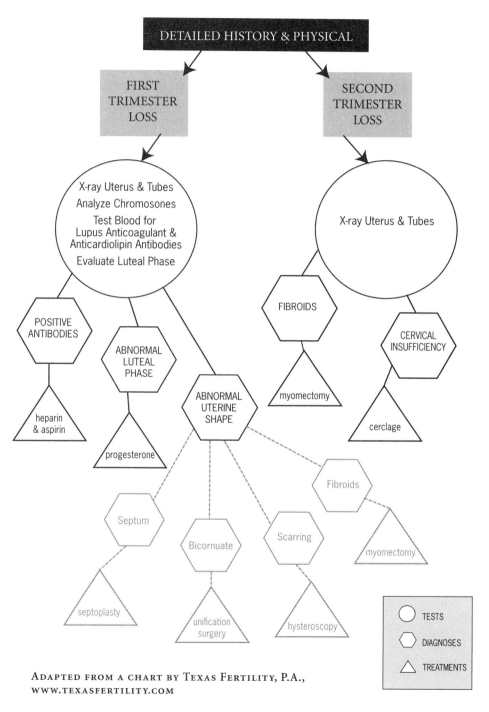

ADAPTED FROM A CHART BY TEXAS FERTILITY, P.A.,
WWW.TEXASFERTILITY.COM

- Glucose tolerance test: This test is often performed during pregnancy, too. It involves drinking a glucose solution and then testing sugar in the blood after one or three hours (usually one hour initially). Elevated glucose levels may suggest diabetes.

- Fasting insulin and glucose: This test identifies the condition known as insulin resistance, in which insulin is elevated and glucose is normal. Insulin resistance can be associated with recurrent miscarriage.

- Homocysteine: High levels of homocysteine are associated with miscarriage. Some practitioners feel that this test is more useful than the MTHFR screening, and others order it only if the MTHFR gene mutation is homozygous (see page 54).

OTHER TESTS

- Fetal karyotype: This test of embryonic or fetal tissue involves analyzing the baby's chromosomes to see if major chromosomal problems caused the miscarriage. Sometimes the cells are not viable and so cannot be analyzed, but usually a karyotype can be determined.

- Hysterosalpingogram (HSG): This test involves injecting dye into the uterus and then X-raying the uterus and fallopian tubes to identify any abnormalities.

- Hysteroscopy and laparoscopy: Some practitioners go straight to one of these tests instead of performing an HSG. The test is done with the woman under local or general anesthesia. The doctor uses a scope to check for abnormalities in the uterus. In a laparoscopy, the scope goes through an incision in the abdomen; in a hysteroscopy, it goes through the cervix.

- Vaginal ultrasound: As part of a miscarriage workup, a vaginal probe is inserted to examine the ovaries and uterus for abnormalities.

- Endometrial biopsy: Usually done in the second half of the menstrual cycle, this test involves taking a sample of the uterine lining to see whether it has developed normally.

- Sperm DNA integrity (SDI): This test evaluates the chromosomes in the male partner's sperm. If the sperm test as having frequently abnormal chromosomes or frequent breaks in the DNA, miscarriage may be more likely.

Receiving the Results

With most miscarriage tests, the results won't be available immediately. You'll go to a lab for a blood draw and maybe have a hysterosalpingogram, and then you'll have to wait until the next appointment with your practitioner to find out if there's anything to treat. The wait can be tough.

Miscarriage testing puts you in the unusual position of hoping, subconsciously or even consciously, to find something wrong with you. You may hope to have a blood-clotting disorder or low progesterone, and your friends and relatives may think you're crazy for thinking this way. But finding a cause for your miscarriages can help you feel you have some control over your situation. You may end up disappointed if the tests find nothing to treat. These feelings are totally normal.

In the days preceding your appointment, make a list of questions for your practitioner. When you're sitting in the office, all the research that you've done and the questions that you have may fly off to your subconscious rather than staying in the forefront of your mind. If you remember them only when you leave the office, you'll kick yourself for not asking your questions. So write them down in advance. Talk to your partner, who I hope can attend the appointments with you, and be sure that you both understand what information you're looking for. Don't be afraid to ask a lot of questions.

You may want to postpone any attempt to conceive during the period that you are waiting for your test results, on the off chance that a problem is found that requires early treatment.

A Note About Self-blame

In the process of looking for a cause of their miscarriages, many women have an unspoken, possibly subconscious fear: Is it my fault that I lost the baby? After all, even the word *miscarriage* seems to imply that the mom carried the baby wrong (although *miscarriage* is better than some alternative terms for pregnancy loss). We may hold onto a deep fear that our miscarriages are our fault even if we know this can't be true. The guilt can be very hard to live with.

With very few exceptions, miscarriage is no one's fault. If you turn out to have a medical problem that caused your losses, you probably couldn't have known about it in advance. Miscarriages usually don't happen because of something a woman does or doesn't do.

> *I felt like my body was broken. What was wrong with me that I couldn't do what every other woman does?*
>
> —PAULA

> *I searched for some sort of meaning for what was happening to us, and the only thing I could come up with is that I was a terrible person who deserved punishment. This is stupid, I know, but at the time I truly believed it.*
>
> —WANDA

> *I felt it was my responsibility to keep the baby growing inside me safe.*
>
> —MERALEE

> *I felt I was less of a woman for not being able to carry a child.*
>
> —JENNIFER

Treatment

This section provides an overview of various miscarriage treatments—what they are, what they do, and how much evidence exists for their efficacy. The following treatments are the most commonly used in today's miscarriage therapy:

- Heparin

- Low-dose aspirin

Author's Story

*I*t isn't reasonable or rational, but I still blame myself for my losses, especially the third one. It was the second cycle in which I was trying to get pregnant following the preceding loss. I had called a reproductive endocrinologist (RE) and had an appointment in two months. In my frustration with the wait, I had also called an OB-GYN who I had heard did a lot of work with infertility. At that time I had a bias toward female practitioners; the OB-GYN was a woman, whereas the RE was a man. So when we got a call saying the RE had an opening for us the following Monday, at the same time as the OB-GYN appointment, I decided to keep the original appointment with the OB-GYN.

I was eight days past ovulation, and I hoped the OB-GYN would be willing to test my progesterone level. This was the only possible miscarriage cause that I hadn't been tested for in the past, as far as I knew. But the doctor, who used the term "habitual abortion," said that she couldn't do anything for me until I'd had three miscarriages. She did, however, order a test for progesterone, and my level did turn out to be low. Although I didn't know it yet, I was pregnant, and I miscarried once more. I kept the later appointment with the RE and never called the OB-GYN again.

I got pregnant with my daughter later on, while taking a high dose of progesterone prescribed by the RE. I'll always wonder if I wouldn't have lost the third baby if I had just taken the earlier appointment with the RE. I remind myself I wouldn't have my daughter now if I hadn't lost the other baby; I can't regret anything about her existence. But I still wonder.

- Progesterone supplements

- Clomid (clomiphene citrate)

- Folic acid and B vitamins

- Prednisone

- Metformin

- Intravenous immunoglobulin

- Paternal leukocyte immunization

- Bromocriptine/cabergoline

- Human chorionic gonadotropin injections

- Preimplantation genetic diagnosis

- Uterine reconstruction

- Cerclage

HEPARIN

This anticoagulant is used to treat a number of blood-clotting and immune disorders, most commonly antiphospholipid syndrome (see page 57). The drug is administered by injection to the abdominal area. A good body of evidence shows that heparin is effective against antiphospholipid syndrome. A meta-analysis published by the well-respected *Cochrane Review* found that heparin, in combination with low-dose aspirin, reduces pregnancy loss by as much as 54 percent, although the researchers also concluded that more trials were needed to compare the effectiveness of different types of heparin. Researchers believe that heparin works by improving the ability of the placenta to properly implant in the uterus and by blocking certain properties of antiphospholipid antibodies.

Heparin is also commonly used to treat other coagulation disorders, such as factor V Leiden, and some practitioners prescribe it for women with elevated homocysteine levels as well, and even for patients with unexplained recurrent miscarriage, just in case it might work. The use of heparin in the absence of coagulation disorders has less solid evidence behind it, although a *Cochrane Review* study concluded that this treatment is worthy of more investigation. A recent study found that heparin even in the absence of coagulation disorders could help improve implantation.

Heparin is a naturally occurring substance found in everyone's body, and it is used by tens of thousands of pregnant women in the United States every year. Ample evidence shows that it causes no defects or bleeding abnormalities in the baby. Nor does heparin contribute to bleeding problems in the pregnant woman, if it is used in the proper dosage. But heparin is not entirely risk-free; it can be allergenic for sensitive individuals, particularly those with a history of asthma or allergies, and because it thins the blood it can exacerbate or cause bleeding disorders if not used very carefully. It may interact with other medications as well.

Heparin has a calcium-depleting effect, so all women who take heparin during pregnancy are advised to take extra calcium as well.

LOW-DOSE ASPIRIN

Although its effectiveness is well documented only for antiphospholipid syndrome, aspirin is also sometimes used as a part of treatment for recurrent miscarriage, in daily doses of 75 to 81 milligrams. The theory is that, because aspirin thins the blood, it should be effective against coagulation disorders.

PROGESTERONE SUPPLEMENTS

Low progesterone levels are associated with miscarriage. In theory, supplemental progesterone prevents miscarriages that are caused by the failure of a woman's body to produce adequate progesterone for what would otherwise be a viable pregnancy. Researchers disagree, however, about whether low progesterone levels cause a pregnancy to be unviable or whether they only indicate that the pregnancy is unviable. The truth probably differs from one situation to the next.

A great deal of research suggests that, for most women, supplemental progesterone does not prevent miscarriage. A meta-analysis published in the *Cochrane Review* found "no evidence to support the routine use of progestogen [progesterone or a drug that mimics its actions] to prevent miscarriage in early to mid pregnancy." As the reviewers reported, 14 separate trials involving 1,988 pregnant women found no statistically significant difference in the rate of successful pregnancies between the women who received progesterone and those who received a placebo or no treatment. Because of this study, many practitioners say there is no evidence that progesterone can prevent miscarriage, although it can delay the onset of a predestined miscarriage.

Just 3 of the 14 trials, however, involved only women who had had *recurrent* miscarriages. These three trials did find that pregnancy outcomes were significantly better among the groups who received progesterone. The reviewers concluded that "further trials in women with a history of recurrent miscarriage may be warranted, given the trend for improved live birth rates in these women and the finding of no statistically significant difference between treatment and control groups in rates of adverse effects suffered by either mother or baby in the available evidence." A 1989 review in the *British Journal of Gynaecology* had similar findings.

To further complicate the issue, many of the trials used not true progesterone but progestins, drugs designed to mimic the natural hormone. "Natural" progesterone supplements, which are identical to the progesterone your body produces, may well behave differently in the body. No one knows for sure; this question has not been adequately studied.

Low progesterone levels may be a root cause of miscarriage for some women. Researchers have postulated that progesterone levels may be lowered because of stress, or problems with the corpus luteum cyst, the site on the ovary that releases progesterone until the placenta is ready to take over (see page 48). Some practitioners prescribe progesterone only to women who have tested as having a luteal-phase defect, as indicated by the day-21 progesterone test (see pages 79). Other practitioners are willing to prescribe progesterone to any women who have had miscarriages, just because it might help. Practitioners who prescribe supplemental progesterone will usually do this only very early in pregnancy.

Studies have found no health risks in taking progesterone supplements in pregnancy. Know that progesterone cannot prevent miscarriages that are caused by chromosomal abnormalities but can only delay bleeding in these cases.

Progesterone comes in five different forms. Your doctor can prescribe a pill that you swallow, an injection, a gel that you apply vaginally, a suppository, or a cream that you rub into your skin. The *Cochrane Review* study found no difference in efficacy according to delivery method. If you have a documented progesterone deficiency, however, it's probably best to use some form of prescription progesterone rather than an over-the-counter type from a health-food store, since it's hard to be sure of the dosage and absorption rate of over-the-counter products. Do look for a

There likely are some people whom progesterone therapy helps, but there's never been a well-done trial that shows benefit. Progesterone therapy may help a good pregnancy and will definitely prolong a bad pregnancy. At the end of the day, there's no harm but possible benefit. We give progesterone under that premise—that we're not going to hurt anyone. I believe that the majority of people I give progesterone to don't need it, but they want to know that they're doing everything they can. If it does no harm, makes me and them feel better, and makes sure there's enough progesterone around, let's do it. We do a lot of other things under that premise.

—MARK P. LEONDIRES, M.D., F.A.C.O.G.

For women who have a clearly short luteal phase, progesterone is indicated. If the second part of the cycle is of normal length, then probably there is no need. The decision is based on each individual patient. You cannot say yes or no for all. A subgroup of women may benefit but probably not everyone. It's very controversial.

— PAOLO RINAUDO, M.D., PH.D.

Many OB-GYNs have guessed that some women do not make enough progesterone to support an early pregnancy. Although this seems to be unusual, I believe it may, on some occasions, be responsible for pregnancy loss. In a few of my patients I have been able to find no other cause for repetitive loss except low progesterone levels in early pregnancy. I supplemented them with progesterone, and their pregnancies were successful. Did I really help with the progesterone? I don't know! I will, however, take the credit.

—BARRY JACOBS, M.D., F.A.C.O.G

"natural" progesterone that is "bioidentical" to what your body produces; your doctor can give you more information on this.

*I am using natural progesterone cream to combat the low proges-
terone I suspect I have, but my doctor is not quite on board.*

—Abigail

*The next time I get pregnant, if my levels are low, I will be given
progesterone vaginal suppositories. I am not looking forward to that,
but if it helps to avoid another loss, sign me up! I'd even do the shots
every day!*

—Kimberly

*We tried natural progesterone suppositories, but probably too late. I
knew there was only a slim chance that these might work, but I was
willing to try anything.*

—A. J.

*I used progesterone suppositories, but they only kept a failing preg-
nancy from failing completely. I would have miscarried at 6 weeks
instead of 11 weeks if I hadn't used the suppositories.*

—Wendy

CLOMID (CLOMIPHENE CITRATE)

This drug is also occasionally prescribed for women who have had recurrent miscarriages with luteal-phase defect. It is taken before pregnancy,
in the first week of the menstrual cycle.

Prescribing Clomid for luteal-phase defect has a number of different
supporting rationales. Some women have been told that Clomid reduces
the odds of miscarriage by causing the release of multiple eggs, and
thereby increases the odds that a viable pregnancy will result during a
particular cycle. Another explanation is that Clomid produces a stronger
corpus luteum (see page 48).

Only a few studies, however, have found that Clomid can reduce miscarriage rates. Some studies have actually found higher rates of miscar-

Author's Story

With my third miscarriage, I got a progesterone test done at eight days past ovulation. The doctor said the level was normal, but I knew from my online research that it was quite low for a cycle that involved pregnancy. I talked the doctor into prescribing progesterone suppositories, but I ended up miscarrying anyway. I later learned that the suppositories she prescribed were of a quite low dosage.

The next time I got pregnant, I was seeing a reproductive endocrinologist (RE). I again had a progesterone test, and the level was lower than it was supposed to be (but higher than it had been with the previous pregnancy). The RE gave me oral progesterone in a much higher dosage than before. He rechecked my progesterone level and raised the dosage twice before the level was where it should be. I took progesterone all through the first trimester, and the pregnancy resulted in my daughter. I suppose I'll never know if the progesterone was the key to my finally having a successful pregnancy.

riage following Clomid use, although the results may have been skewed by preexisting conditions in the study participants. It's worth considering, also, that by stimulating the release of multiple eggs Clomid increases the chance of multiple births, which are riskier to the mother's health. For these reasons, Clomid is seldom prescribed for recurrent miscarriage alone, without associated problems such as difficulty getting pregnant or polycystic ovarian syndrome (see page 50).

FOLIC ACID AND B VITAMINS

You probably have come across the recommendation that all women of childbearing age should consume plenty of folic acid, or folate. Supplementation with this nutrient can drastically decrease neural-tube defects such as spina bifida and devastating disorders like anencephaly. Because research also links folate deficiency to miscarriage, many practitioners recommend extra folate supplements for patients who have experienced recurrent miscarriage, especially those with the homozygous MTHFR mutation (see page 54), which is associated with folate deficiency.

Extra B vitamins along with extra folate are often suggested for reducing high homocysteine levels, which have been associated with an increased risk of miscarriage (see page 54).

Vitamin B_{12} deficiency has been independently correlated with higher miscarriage rates, although the reasons for this correlation are not yet well understood. Women following a vegan diet may be at greater risk for vitamin B_{12} deficiency, since it comes primarily from animal-derived foods (vegetarians who consume dairy products and eggs should not lack for this vitamin). Taking extra B vitamins and folic acid, in moderate dosages, does not appear to carry any risks and may in fact be beneficial, but discuss this treatment with your practitioner before trying it.

PREDNISONE

This corticosteroid is commonly used to treat a variety of immune disorders, particularly those related to inflammation. It can have unpleasant side effects with long-term use, including headaches, mood changes, weight gain, acne, hair growth, elevated blood pressure, fatigue, and sweating, to name a few. Yet prednisone can be powerfully effective when its use is merited. Some high-risk specialists treat women with lupus or other autoimmune disorders with prednisone to prevent flare-ups during pregnancy, and many reproductive immunology clinics use prednisone to prevent miscarriages thought to be associated with autoimmune disease. Any corticosteroid use during pregnancy may be risky, however. These drugs can cause high blood pressure, gestational diabetes, preterm delivery, low birth weight, increased bone loss in the mother (especially when used in combination with heparin), and possibly long-term adrenal suppression. The use of prednisone in pregnant women specifically to prevent miscarriage should probably be viewed as experimental.

METFORMIN

Also known by the trade name Glucophage, this drug is most commonly prescribed for patients with type 2 diabetes to reduce blood sugar. Some studies have shown that metformin may also reduce miscarriage rates for women with polycystic ovarian syndrome (PCOS, see page 50). Overall, the drug appears to be safe in pregnancy, and for this reason many practitioners prescribe it to miscarriage patients who they feel may benefit from it. Others, more cautious, say that metformin should be used only in clinical trials until its safety record and efficacy are better established.

> *My reproductive endocrinologist was very honest about Glucophage use for PCOS being "off-label" but said that he had had very good results in the past with its use to help prevent miscarriage in PCOS women. He provided me with several articles and studies showing a decrease in risk of miscarriage.*
>
> —MICHELLE

INTRAVENOUS IMMUNOGLOBULIN (IVIG)

This is a human blood product containing pooled antibodies. It's commonly used to treat a variety of immune-system disorders, and some reproductive immunology clinics use it to treat immunological causes of recurrent miscarriage. This use of IVIg is highly controversial. A few studies have found it to be beneficial for carefully screened patients who have evidence of immune abnormalities, but most double-blind studies of unscreened miscarriage patients have found it to have no benefit beyond that of a placebo. It remains to be seen whether IVIg will ultimately play a role in recurrent-miscarriage treatment. Remember that, because IVIg is a blood product, it carries at least a theoretical risk of HIV or hepatitis transmission.

Regarding IVIg and paternal leukocyte immunizations, there is a subgroup of women who could theoretically benefit from these treatments. But until they are proven to work, I would not use them. The evidence is not there, and they are expensive. Until studies can show some difference in success rates between these treatments and a placebo, these treatments are not recommended.

— PAOLO RINAUDO, M.D., PH.D.

PATERNAL LEUKOCYTE IMMUNIZATION

This is probably one of the strangest-sounding miscarriage therapies available. It involves injecting white blood cells from the father into the mother to induce her body to make the appropriate blocking antibodies. A *Cochrane Review* study deemed the treatment (and other immuno-therapy treatments for recurrent miscarriage) to provide "no significant beneficial effect over placebo in improving the live birth rate." But as with IVIg, studies that use screening tools to distinguish who needs the treatment and who does not generally meet with better success. For now the treatment is still experimental, and time will tell whether it has a role in miscarriage treatment.

BROMOCRIPTINE/CABERGOLINE

These drugs are used to treat a variety of diseases, including Parkinson's. Both have been used with some success to reduce prolactin levels in women with hyperprolactinemia (see page 51) and to improve their pregnancy outcomes.

HUMAN CHORIONIC
GONADOTROPIN INJECTIONS

As discussed in chapter 1, human chorionic gonadotropin, or hCG, is a characteristic hormone of pregnancy (see page 5). In an experimental treatment for certain hormonal disorders associated with miscarriage, women have been given supplemental hCG, and in a few trials this has met with some success. The evidence, however, is considered too preliminary to justify widespread use of hCG in this manner.

PREIMPLANTATION GENETIC DIAGNOSIS (PGD)

With this technique, used in conjunction with in vitro fertilization, a cell from the developing embryo is extracted and analyzed for common chromosomal abnormalities. PGD is expensive and still under development, but it appears to be an excellent therapy for couples who miscarry repeatedly because of an increased tendency toward chromosomal abnormalities. As the technology improves, the technique should become even better for screening embryos.

PGD has been the subject of controversy; some people see it as a way of creating "designer babies." Whether or not you agree, you may be discouraged by its great expense, which is rarely covered by medical insurance, and by the fact that it has to be combined with in vitro fertilization. As an alternative, some women who have experienced recurrent miscarriage due to chromosomal problems, as well as women who have few eggs left in their ovaries, choose to use donor eggs or sperm. This option allows many couples who otherwise could not to experience pregnancy and birth.

UTERINE RECONSTRUCTION

For women who have been diagnosed with certain types of anatomical problems, such as a uterine septum, the recommended treatment may be surgery. This involves checking into a hospital and undergoing anesthesia (usually general anesthesia) and having the uterine problem corrected in conjunction with hysteroscopy or laparoscopy (see page 82). Like any surgery, uterine reconstruction carries some risks, and you should discuss them with your doctor before proceeding. But reconstruction appears to improve pregnancy outcomes for women with uterine abnormalities (see page 40).

A uterine septum is treated by hysteroscopic resection of the septum. This is a surgery that people need to take seriously, because you have to be careful that you don't go too far.
—MARK P. LEONDIRES, M.D., F.A.C.O.G.

CERCLAGE

This controversial treatment for cervical insufficiency is performed to hold the cervix closed when it begins to dilate early or, in women who have miscarried, to prevent premature dilation.

There are three types of cervical cerclage. In a McDonald cerclage, a band suture is placed in the upper portion of the cervix and then is removed at about the thirty-seventh week of pregnancy. A Shirodkar cerclage is similar to a McDonald cerclage but is placed in the wall of the uterus and is intended to be permanent, necessitating a cesarean delivery. An abdominal cerclage, which involves stitching the cervix through the abdomen, is the least common of the three procedures.

The value of cervical cerclage may depend on multiple factors that vary by the individual woman's circumstances. Some studies have found no proof that cerclage prevents pregnancy loss, whereas others have found that it offers benefit. It's likely that the success or failure depends heavily on the technique used and the circumstances, such as whether cerclage is used as an emergency treatment when the cervix dilates prematurely or as an elective, preventive treatment in women with a history of second-trimester pregnancy loss. One smaller study saw great benefit in treating women with recurrent miscarriage with cerclage early in the second trimester, before any sign of premature dilation.

Supportive Care

If you've had testing for the miscarriage causes generally accepted by the medical community and found nothing to treat, you have another option that has been increasingly shown to help prevent miscarriage: Find a supportive practitioner. Frequent tests, round-the-clock access to a physician, and ample reassurance make up a treatment plan practitioners call TLC, or tender loving care. Studies have found that, for women who have ruled out known causes of miscarriage, TLC produces better pregnancy outcomes than standard prenatal care. Having a supportive practitioner might be more important than you'd initially think!

I think that TLC is an important part of stress management. Patients need to realize that there is help for them out there, and that the majority are able to go on and have a healthy, happy pregnancy.

—MARK P. LEONDIRES, M.D., F.A.C.O.G.

Surrogacy

Pregnancy loss is hard on the soul. If you've tried everything, you've ruled out chromosomal issues, and your heart just can't take another miscarriage, surrogacy may be an option. Surrogacy starts with in vitro fertilization, but the embryos are transferred into a surrogate mother, who carries one or more babies through pregnancy. The practice is controversial, but most women who volunteer themselves as surrogates have had children of their own and report the surrogacy experience as positive. Surrogacy has brought hope to some people who would have otherwise had none. One medical journal published a case study of a woman who had 24 consecutive miscarriages before finally becoming a mother through surrogacy. Appendix B lists resources for investigating this option. (Don't forget to consider adoption; Appendix B also suggests some resources for this.)

I've tried to cover all the important miscarriage treatments in this chapter, including the most common experimental ones. If you search for more information on the Internet, though, you may read of a treatment not mentioned herein. If you have a practitioner whom you trust, discuss the treatment and its pros and cons. Ask whether there's a chance the treatment might help you and, even if it's unproven, whether it might pose any risk at all to your baby. If the answer to the latter question is no, then the worst that can happen if you try the treatment is that it won't make a difference. At least you won't have to wonder forever after if it would have worked.

I hope that with the information in this chapter you'll be able to work with your practitioner to develop a plan for testing and, if needed, treatment for the causes of your miscarriages. Your complete evaluation can probably be finished in five to six weeks. During this time you and your partner should not try to conceive. Your physician will ask you to wait until all the tests have been performed and a treatment plan has been developed, and possibly longer (see chapter 6).

All the waiting, before trying to conceive again and between ovulation periods once you start trying, can drive you batty—especially when you're still grieving the loss of your previous pregnancy. In the next chapter, we'll discuss things you can do on your own to reduce stress and get through this difficult time with your sanity intact.

CHAPTER 4

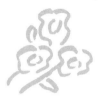

Alternative Treatments and Stress Reduction

THE PHRASE *ALTERNATIVE TREATMENT* means different things to different people. Some people distrust conventional medicine and turn to alternative treatment as a first line of therapy for any health problem encountered. Others hear the phrase and automatically think of snake oil and treatments that are a colossal waste of money and have no effect proven by science.

The truth is that some alternative treatments have a strong base in science, and many alternative therapies have been shown by studies to be beneficial for treating a variety of health conditions. The problem is that alternative medicine is a lot harder to study than conventional medicine, because most alternative practitioners and therapies treat the entire person rather than only specific symptoms; this is what the term *holistic medicine* means.

For example, if you ask a conventional practitioner what to do about a headache you'll likely be told to take a Tylenol. If you're lucky, the Tylenol will suppress the pain so you no longer have a headache. But if you ask a holistic practitioner what to do about a headache, he or she will probably ask you questions about the level of stress in your life, whether you've had enough water to drink that day, whether you sleep on an adequate mattress at night, and so on. The holistic practitioner looks for the reason that you have a headache in the first place rather than merely for a way you can get rid of the headache. And if the practitioner concludes that your headaches are caused by stress and recommends a series of lifestyle changes to decrease stress, and if your headaches then go away, it's harder to judge exactly what caused you to stop having headaches than it would be if you just took a Tylenol and the headache went away. But, if making the lifestyle changes does indeed cause the headaches to stop, it's better in the long run to have made these changes than to pop a Tylenol every time you get a headache, because the Tylenol does nothing to address the cause of the problem.

Holistic medicine often turns people off prematurely, for a number of reasons. Some alternative practitioners take a "New Age" approach; they talk about the mind-body connection and spiritual healing in a way that doesn't appeal to everyone. In addition, because there are so many self-proclaimed "holistic" practitioners out there using self-invented methods with no scientific evidence behind them and peddling miracle cures for large sums of money, sometimes perception of the entire field is tainted. It's important to be aware that not all alternative practitioners are licensed, and that even many licensed practitioners may not be covered by your medical insurance. But slowly this is changing; more and more insurance providers are covering such services as acupuncture and chiropractic treatments. At the time of this writing, moreover, naturopathic doctors are licensed as primary-care providers in 19 states.

Alternative Medicine and Miscarriages

Holistic medicine can have a place in miscarriage treatment, particularly in the area of stress management. With studies starting to tie stress and anxiety to increased risk of miscarriage or difficulty conceiving, taking care of yourself as an entire person and not just as a uterus seems more important than ever. For this reason, this chapter will not only discuss alternative treatments that may boost your odds of a successful pregnancy, but it will also offer suggestions about how you can reduce the stress in your life and better cope with the emotions surrounding your miscarriages. These are the topics we'll discuss:

- Dietary changes

- Nutritional supplements

- Acupuncture

- Herbal medicine

- Weight loss

- Yoga and meditation

- Homeopathy

Watch out for anyone who makes unrealistic claims about what a particular therapy can do, and steer clear of anyone who promises a total cure.

But don't let the bad apples mar your opinion of the entire alternative-medicine field. To be sure the person you're seeing is qualified, check his or her credentials against a national certifying body, and watch out for people who have obtained credentials through mail-order degree mills. For example, a naturopathic doctor (N.D.) who attended Bastyr University in Seattle (or another similar naturopathic medical school) will have undergone training of a similar caliber to that of a medical doctor (M.D.), but some practitioners who call themselves N.D.'s have gotten their degrees from a diploma mill and have no formal clinical training. Certifying bodies exist for most holistic specialties, to assure a certain level of quality in practice.

A growing number of medical studies have demonstrated that "natural" or "complementary" medicine significantly improves conception and pregnancy success rates. If length of use is an indicator of usefulness, then I offer that Oriental medicine, at about 3,500 years of continuous practice (for countless millions of individuals), may be considered efficacious.

—GERALD WILLIAMS, L.AC. (CALIFORNIA),
D.A. (RHODE ISLAND), M.S.T.O.M.

Alternative Treatments and Stress Reduction

DIETARY CHANGES

I've never seen a whit of proof that eating or not eating particular foods causes a woman to miscarry. Some studies correlate obesity with miscarriage, but the link is not well understood, and the miscarriages are probably caused not by overeating but rather by associated hormonal problems. I have seen reports that say maintaining a healthy diet makes a person feel better and more energetic, and that can't be a bad thing when you're trying to make a baby. Let's look at a few of these studies:

* In a study of 149 men and 156 women, psychology researchers from the State University of New York found that participants who followed a cholesterol-lowering diet reported reductions in aggression and depression during the course of the diet.

* Researchers from the University of Athens, in Greece, found that following a "Mediterranean" diet, high in unsaturated fats and complex carbohydrates, reduced inflammation, C-reactive protein, homocysteine, and other cardiovascular markers. (Remember, these factors may also play a role in miscarriage.)

* Researchers in Dublin, Ireland, found that a "Mediterranean" diet could also have a beneficial effect on insulin sensitivity in people with type 2 diabetes.

* A Swedish study of more than 59,000 women found that diets high in fruits, vegetables, whole grains, fish, and low-fat dairy products reduced the risk of death from cancer and cardiovascular disease.

* As reported in the *New England Journal of Medicine*, a study that followed 84,941 female nurses for 16 years found that a healthy diet could prevent type 2 diabetes about half the time.

And that's just a few of many. You cannot go wrong in opting for nutrient-rich fruits and vegetables over potato chips, fast food, and other highly processed foods.

NUTRITIONAL SUPPLEMENTS

We head into murkier territory as we consider the value of nutritional supplements for women who have experienced miscarriage. There is much conflicting evidence about the efficacy of vitamin and mineral supplements. Some claim they're worthless; others claim they're the greatest thing since sliced bread, if not greater than sliced bread. The truth is probably somewhere in between and notoriously difficult to determine.

Studies of nutritional supplements may be unreliable because the nutrients in different formulations may be absorbed by the body differently. So, for example, if you examine the overall health of a large group of people who claim to have taken a vitamin C supplement every day for the past six months, you have to take into account that some of them might have chosen a type of vitamin C that wasn't very absorbable by the body. Vitamin C can take the form of ascorbic acid, sodium ascorbate, calcium ascorbate, potassium ascorbate, or another compound, and there is inadequate research to say whether all these compounds behave the same way in the body.

In addition, absorption of some nutrients in the body may depend on the availability of other nutrients, from dietary sources, supplements, or both. For example, people who are deficient in vitamin D may not absorb calcium well.

Accurate studies of nutritional supplements must control participants' food intake. The people in a vitamin C study may have consumed varying amounts of vitamin C in their diets. It is hard to make nutritional comparisons among groups of people outside a clinical setting, and even within a clinical setting it is difficult to control the diets of groups of people for any meaningful length of time.

A *Cochrane Review* study of vitamin supplementation and miscarriages found no difference in miscarriage rates between women taking vitamin supplements and women not taking them. But the study, which looked at "17 trials assessing supplementation with any vitamin(s) starting prior to 20 weeks' gestation," did not differentiate among specific vitamin combinations or dosages or conduct laboratory analysis to verify whether the women were absorbing the vitamin supplements. A few studies have shown associations between miscarriage and specific nutritional deficiencies (for example, selenium), so a logical assumption would be that women who have nutritional deficiencies ought to take supplements or attempt dietary changes to raise levels of the deficient nutrients (although the problem may be poor absorption rather than low intake). Scattered studies have found beneficial effects from specific types of vitamin supplementation; for example, one study found that vitamin C supplementation improved progesterone levels. But few of the existing studies are able to account for all potentially confounding factors.

For this reason, too, the potential for harm from nutritional supplements, especially in megadoses, is not well understood. Vitamin A is a good example; studies in the 1950s and 1960s linked megadoses of vitamin A with birth defects, but the link is still not well understood. Doctors typically advise women to avoid excessive vitamin A in pregnancy, to be on the safe side.

Except for the issue of folic acid and neural-tube defects, the effects of nutritional supplements on pregnancy have not been studied adequately enough for practitioners to make solid recommendations. To reduce the risk of birth defects, however, it's a good idea to take a daily prenatal multivitamin, regular multivitamin, or folic-acid supplement beginning three months before conception. See page 194 for advice on selecting a prenatal vitamin.

ACUPUNCTURE

This medical practice, which involves applying special needles to very specific points in the body, is more than 2,000 years old. Acupuncture originated in China and has recently become a mainstream therapy in the United States, where a survey found that more than 8.2 million adults have used acupuncture as a treatment. How acupuncture works, exactly, is not well studied, but the traditional theory is that applying the needles promotes healing by changing the body's flow of energy.

If this sounds strange to you, you're not alone, but don't write off acupuncture as quackery too quickly. Studies have documented that it may work in treating some conditions, particularly chronic pain, headache, and alcoholism. But the efficacy of acupuncture is difficult to study, because it is nearly impossible to design a double-blind study (one in which a placebo group is compared to an experimental group, and neither participants nor practitioners know who is in which group) with accurately matched groups. Skeptics allege that the benefits of acupuncture are psychological, but if the treatment helps reduce stress and this reduction results in healing, might that not be a good enough reason to use acupuncture?

Many women have tried acupuncture as a treatment for recurrent miscarriage, and some swear that this is the reason that they finally carried a baby to term. A few scattered studies have linked acupuncture to a reduced incidence of miscarriage, but the results have not been definitive, because it's impossible to say whether acupuncture, chance, stress relief, or some other factor resulted in the successful pregnancies. Acupuncture is very safe, however, so consider it as a treatment that couldn't hurt and might help.

Many alternative or complementary therapies—including meditation, exercise, massage, yoga, gardening, prayer, and acupuncture—have shown benefit in treating not only recurrent pregnancy loss but other medical problems as well. The common link between these beneficial activities is stress reduction, or both mental and physical relaxation. Pushing a particular therapy to an extreme, however, is probably not beneficial.

— WILLIAM H. KUTTEH M.D., PH.D., H.C.L.D.

HERBAL MEDICINE

Like nutritional supplements, herbs are one of the more common alternative treatments for health problems. Remember that herbs (and other natural substances) are the basis for some prescription drugs, and that they can have powerful effects on the body, so you cannot assume that they are safe merely because they are natural. Some common herbal therapies carry significant safety risks; some can even induce a miscarriage or cause birth defects.

That said, herbal medicine may certainly have the power to do good. Some herbs may improve the chance of conception or reduce miscarriage risks by boosting progesterone levels. Herbalists commonly cite false unicorn root (also called starwort, fairy wand, *Chamaelirium luteum, Helonias dioica, Helonias lutea,* and *Veratrum luteum*) as having the power to reduce a woman's chance of miscarriage. If you want to pursue herbal therapy, however, you need to understand that the majority of medicinal herbs have not undergone rigorous testing for safety and efficacy, and they are probably best used under the supervision of a licensed naturopathic physician or a member of the American Herbalists Guild who has undergone a training program certified by the guild. You should also be sure to obtain any herbal remedies from a reputable supplier, such as a trusted herbalist.

There are herbs that women have used for a long time to help reduce infertility due to recurrent miscarriage. If a woman is going to miscarry, sometimes herbs will help encourage uterine contractions and make the process easier. Paradoxically, if the threatened miscarriage is not inevitable, the herbs will help maintain the pregnancy.

As you would expect, every practitioner has his or her favorite herb or combination of herbs. Herbs purported to affect miscarriage risks include wild yam *(Dioscorea villosa)*, cramp bark *(Viburnum opulus)*, partridge berry *(Mitchella repens)*, red raspberry leaf *(Rubus idaeus)*, black cohosh *(Cimicifuga racemosa)*, black haw *(Viburnum prunifolium)*, and false unicorn root *(Chamaelirium luteum)*.

The effects of herbs on hormonal balance are not clear and have not been clinically demonstrated, to my knowledge. But there seems to be significant anecdotal and experiential evidence that suggests their effectiveness. Some herbs are said to have an "estrogenic effect," which does not mean that they contain estrogen. Instead, their chemical structure matches estrogen receptors in the body, and so they mimic the effects of estrogen. When there is an imbalance in the system, some herbs, especially chasteberry *(Vitex agnus-castus)*, red clover *(Trifolium pratense)*, and false unicorn root *(Chamaelirium luteum)*, help bring the body back into balance.

Stress and anxiety are contributing factors to persistent infertility. Stress in the form of toxic overload, as well as emotional and mental stress, can reduce fertility. Often one of the first things herbalists recommend for women having difficulty conceiving is a thorough detoxification, using herbs to clear the body of chemical pollutants stored in the tissues. Our bodies are very capable of rebalancing themselves when they are not burdened by an overload of toxins. This is also an important time to reevaluate our lifestyles, our level of exercise, even the water we drink and the air we breathe. Good cleansing herbs are licorice root *(Glycyrrhiza glabra)*, burdock root *(Arctium lappa)*, dandelion root *(Taraxacum officinale)*, bupleurum root *(Radix bupleuri)*, yellow dock root *(Rumex crispus)*, red clover *(Trifolium pratense)*, turmeric *(Curcuma longa)*, and milk thistle *(Silybum marianum)*.

Adaptogenic herbs help reduce anxiety and irritability and increase resistance to the effects of stress on the body. They reduce the intensity of the "fight-or-flight" response and increase the body's ability to resist stressors and to come back into balance more readily. Adaptogenic herbs include Siberian ginseng *(Eleutherococcus senticosus)*, schisandra *(Schisandra chinensis)*, ashwagandha *(Withania somnifera)*, reishi mushroom *(Ganoderma lucidum)*, holy basil *(Ocimum sanctum)*, golden root *(Rhodiola rosea)*, and American ginseng *(Panax quinquefolius)*.

In addition to these, there are several naturally calming, or nervine, herbs to help soothe the body and reduce anxiety. These are some nervine herbs: oatstraw *(Avena sativa)*, skullcap *(Scutellaria lateriflora)*, passion flower *(Passiflora incarnata)*, German chamomile *(Matricaria recutita)*, lemon balm *(Melissa officinalis)*, black cohosh *(Cimicifuga racemosa)*, black haw *(Viburnum prunifolium)*, red clover *(Trifolium pratense)*, and lavender *(Lavandula officinalis)*. Meditation, yoga, exercise, and visualization also help with relaxing, letting go, and allowing our bodies to do what they innately know how to do.

—MELINDA OLSON, R.N., B.S.N., COFOUNDER, PRESIDENT, AND MAMA IN CHARGE, EARTH MAMA ANGEL BABY HERBAL-PRODUCTS COMPANY

WEIGHT LOSS

Body weight is a very sensitive subject. I object as much as anyone to the idea that one body type should be universally associated with beauty and femininity, and I am all for the idea of women accepting themselves for who they are and not dwelling on how much they weigh. That said, carrying excess body weight may harm your health by altering the hormonal balance in your body, and may thereby increase your risk of miscarriage (see page 64). Some doctors recommend weight reduction as a part of the treatment plan for women with polycystic ovarian syndrome (PCOS, see page 50) or other hormonal conditions. For these reasons, I want to discuss weight loss as something else you may want to consider to reduce your miscarriage risk and improve your overall health.

Some patients tell me they have friends who weigh much more than they do and who have had successful pregnancies, and this is true. However, miscarriage may occur through a complicated interrelationship of different factors, and obesity may be a contributing factor.

— WILLIAM H. KUTTEH M.D., PH.D., H.C.L.D.

Currently, the body mass index (BMI) is the most common way to judge whether or not a person is underweight, at normal weight, overweight, or obese. BMI is calculated with the following formula:

(BODY WEIGHT IN POUNDS) X 703 / (HEIGHT IN INCHES SQUARED)

A BMI under 25 is considered the target. A person with a BMI of 25 to 30 is considered overweight, and someone with a BMI above 30 is considered obese. A person with a BMI less than 20 is considered underweight.

If your BMI indicates that you are obese, losing some weight might help you get pregnant again more quickly and reduce your risk of miscarriage, and might also reduce your subsequent risk of preeclampsia and other pregnancy complications. Weight reduction should be effected through lifestyle changes (including a healthy diet, exercise, and stress reduction) rather than through crash diets or temporary measures. Keep in mind that crash diets, by depriving your body of needed nutrients, could do more harm than good.

Do not attempt to lose weight if you are currently pregnant.

I worry that my current weight makes my body unable to carry a baby. I'm 30 pounds heavier than when I had my daughter five years ago.

—WENDY

Author's Story

I was borderline obese during the time that my miscarriages took place. Before I got pregnant with my daughter, I lost 20 pounds. I don't know whether losing weight helped me avoid miscarrying again, but I do think it made me feel better about myself and improved my health. I have lost even more weight since that time.

Weight loss can be a major struggle. I think that some people who are overweight get that way because of an almost addictive relationship to food. When I was at my heaviest, food affected me like drugs. If I had certain foods in the house, I would sit and think about them nonstop until I had eaten them all. I could not just grab a handful of chips and put the rest away; I had to eat the entire bag at once. If I did manage to put the bag away, I would sit and think about it being in the cabinet, until I found myself holding the bag and grabbing another handful of chips. This would continue until the bag was empty. Sometimes I even rationalized to myself that I might as well go ahead and eat all the chips in one sitting to get rid of the annoying temptation. It took a while for me to accept that the only thing that would work was to never buy the bag of chips in the first place.

I don't believe in quick-fix diets. I have never heard of an instance in which someone was able to follow a short-term "fad" diet and then resume former unhealthy eating habits and keep the weight off. To lose weight for the long term, you have to make a permanent lifestyle change. For me, what worked was eliminating the trigger foods from my diet, and my house, entirely. I stopped buying them; I kept them away to protect myself from myself. Even today, for me, ordering a pizza or buying a

CONTINUED

roll of Starburst candy or a bag of potato chips would be like opening a Pandora's box. It's much easier to stay away from these things completely than to eat just a little bit of them.

Once I had eliminated the trigger foods, I started counting calories. I picked a number of calories that I felt I likely used in one day to maintain my weight, and then I tried to limit my consumption to 200 calories less than that. I soon began losing weight, and since then I have lost more than 50 pounds and kept it off. I'm able to eat foods that taste good, not just salads and Slim-Fast shakes. If I know I want something with more calories for dinner, I try to eat less earlier in the day. I also limit my consumption of sugars and other processed carbohydrates, because I've found that these foods trigger cravings. I drink a lot of nutrient-rich protein shakes, eat lots of fruits and vegetables, and no longer feel the slightest inclination toward unhealthy foods like candy and potato chips as long as they are not in the house.

Changing unhealthy eating habits doesn't take a lot of time, and exercise is not a requirement for weight loss, although it's good for you and should be a part of your life, if possible. I confess I still do not exercise regularly myself, although I know I should.

If you're considering losing weight, it may help to find a support group, whether in person or online. Having other people to talk with will help you hold yourself to a higher standard. Again, don't pick a fad diet and expect to make a short-term commitment before resuming your old habits. Plan to make a real commitment to your own long-term health.

A fter working with patients for many years, I've found these keys to weight loss: (1) some form of calorie counting, (2) identifying and eliminating problem foods, (3) daily assessment of weight, and (4) lifestyle changes. The problem with most diets is that people go on and off them. Success in weight loss involves identifying and acknowledging problem areas and making permanent changes to correct them.

— WILLIAM H. KUTTEH M.D., PH.D., H.C.L.D.

YOGA AND MEDITATION

M ind-body interventions (such as meditation and yoga) are good general stress relievers.

—MADELINE LICKER FEINGOLD, PH.D., CLINICAL PSYCHOLOGIST
SPECIALIZING IN REPRODUCTIVE MEDICINE, BERKELEY, CALIFORNIA

Meditation isn't just about thinking of nothing and saying "om." The first definition of the verb *meditate* in my Merriam-Webster's dictionary is "to engage in contemplation or reflection." There is no right or wrong way to do this. One person might meditate by sitting in a dark room, staring at a candle, and chanting, while another might take a quiet walk in the woods. Meditation is really about clearing and refreshing your mind.

Meditation actually relieves stress symptoms, according to scientific studies. In fact, specific meditation techniques may provide immense health benefits. Following are some examples of meditation techniques with proven health benefits (keep in mind that I am not endorsing any specific meditation program):

* In an eight-week study at the University of California, Irvine, participants in a mindfulness meditation program reported significantly increased feelings of control in their lives and reductions in psychological symptoms.

* A team of researchers compared participants in mindfulness meditation training to a control group and found that the meditation program brought demonstrable positive effects on brain and immune function.

* A team of researchers found that four months of transcendental meditation helped in normalizing hormonal responses to stress.

* Thai researchers demonstrated that Buddhist meditation could reduce cortisol levels and improve cardiac risk factors.

Are you convinced yet? If not, check out these findings about yoga, a discipline involving meditative stretching and relaxation:

- A 1984 study that examined yoga as a treatment for hypertensive patients found that 65 percent of those practicing yoga were able to manage their hypertension without medication of any kind.

- New York researchers who compared the benefits of yoga and swimming found that yoga participants experienced more improvement in mood than either swimmers or a control group who performed neither exercise.

- Indian researchers found that a year of regular yoga practice could reverse cardiovascular disease.

Stress has more of an influence on health than you might initially think, and you can't go wrong by practicing meditation, yoga, tai chi, or another meditative technique or gentle, relaxing exercise. By building deep relaxation into your day-to-day routine, you can only boost your odds of a successful pregnancy when you conceive again, and you stand a good chance of improving your overall health while you're at it.

Stress affects us, and in early pregnancy there is a delicate balance of hormones and physical response and lots of things that have to happen perfectly. It tends to make some sense that you need to try to manage your own stress. Blaming yourself makes you even more stressed. You need to build into your week two to three hours for yourself for stress release. I encourage all patients with recurrent pregnancy loss to consider some kind of stress relief for themselves, whether that is massage therapy, acupuncture, or prayer—whatever they want to do.

—MARK P. LEONDIRES, M.D., F.A.C.O.G.

HOMEOPATHY

This form of medicine is based on the idea that substances that cause symptoms of illness when administered to healthy people will alleviate similar symptoms when administered to people who are sick. This might sound kooky at first, but numerous studies have shown homeopathy to be beneficial. Naysayers attribute any benefit of homeopathy to the placebo effect, but the placebo effect can't explain the numerous studies that have shown homeopathy to be beneficial in nonhuman animals or in newborn babies, neither of whom are aware that they are being treated. Many write off these studies as being improperly performed, but, since homeopathic remedies are individualized according to the person's particular symptoms, it's nearly impossible to test homeopathic remedies in large, controlled, double-blind studies.

Another reason that so many are skeptical of homeopathy is because, if it works, it works by some method that science cannot yet explain. The most potent homeopathic remedies are diluted to the point that they no longer contain even a molecule of the original substance. But not understanding how something works does not mean that it does *not* work. After all, researchers have yet to understand the reasons that some common prescription drugs work.

At the very least, homeopathy is relatively safe. Studies examining the safety of homeopathy have found that adverse side effects are rather rare and, when they do occur, are not usually serious.

Going Forward

The alternative treatments discussed in this chapter might help you in getting through the experience of miscarriage, but none is right for everyone, and none has been conclusively proven to affect a woman's miscarriage risk. Take them or leave them; they are options for you to choose from as you see fit. Each treatment is sufficiently complex that an entire book might be written to explore it properly, and other people have already written such books. In Appendix B, you'll find recommended resources for each of the treatments discussed here.

A great way to find a good alternative-health specialist is through a support group, in which individuals or couples may have personal recommendations. Also, sometimes open-minded physicians at fertility clinics or OB-GYN offices work with complementary specialists.

—GERALD WILLIAMS, L.AC. (CALIFORNIA),
D.A. (RHODE ISLAND), M.S.T.O.M.

THOUGHTS FOR THE CHILD I LOST

By Sharon Gates

There might come a day sometime in the future
When I don't think about you constantly,
Wonder what you would have looked like,
What color your hair would have been,
And how your smile might have looked.
There might come a day sometime in the future
When I won't wonder what I did wrong.
When I won't blame myself.
When the sharp blade of pain will become dull.
When I can accept this as meant to be.
There might come a day sometime in the future
When I carry another child
And though I will love him beyond measure
And though I will hold him a little tighter,
And though he will be my child,
He won't be you.
There might come a day sometime in the future
When I am happy again.
When I can let go.
When I can look at a baby without aching for you.
But it won't be today.

CHAPTER 5

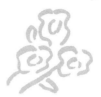

Coping with Pregnancy Loss

I felt as if someone else were living my life and as if I were the body she used. I didn't feel alive.

—TINA

The days seem to enter into slow motion. A minute will feel like half an hour. A half-hour will feel like six hours, and a day will feel like a week. It takes several days and sometimes weeks before anything feels normal.

—JAYNE

I do one task, and then I am exhausted. I never thought I could feel so physically and mentally exhausted. I am trying to work out three times a week to help recover physically and emotionally, but it is so hard, and all I really want to do is curl up in a ball.

—JODY

On the outside I was calm, but if you looked into my eyes you could see the broken pieces of my heart floating around, as if you were looking at shattered glass through a window.

—LISA

*T*HIS HAS GOT TO BE THE HARDEST PART OF MISCARRIAGE: coping with what has happened. How do you do it? How do you find your way back to the world when it feels as if your whole future has been ripped away from you, your heart torn out and put through a shredder, and your body run over by a tank? Your practitioner may shrug his or her shoulders and tell you to try again, but you know it's not that easy. Your friends and family may greet your news with insensitive comments that don't help you at all, and, unless you know someone who has miscarried before, you may feel as if you're alone in the world and wonder if there is something wrong with you for feeling the way you do. You might even have a dialogue with yourself in which you wonder if everyone else is right and you really are just being silly for grieving over a baby you never even held in your arms.

The first thing you need to understand about miscarriage is that it's okay to grieve. Don't feel as if you have to justify your grief by comparing your pain to someone else's. No, you never met your baby, and you may even feel that a miscarriage isn't the same as losing an already-born child, but grief is grief, and there are no competitions for permission to feel pain. Trying to suppress your feelings isn't healthy and would only set you up for problems later on. This chapter is about how to find a healthy way to cope with what has happened and move on with your life.

Don't be surprised if you find yourself feeling angry as well as sad or depressed. After all, anger is one of the much-discussed "five stages of grief," a normal part of coping with loss. You might be angry at yourself even though you know that the loss wasn't your fault, or angry at your doctor because of how he or she treated you, or even angry at your spouse or friends and relatives because they just don't understand what you're going through. It's okay to feel this way, as long as you make sure that your feelings aren't getting in the way of your relationships and keeping you from healing.

The Aftermath

For starters, the hormonal crash that happens within your body when you miscarry is similar to the changes that happen after birth and that can lead to postpartum depression. You are battling biology and emotions at the same time! Lament nature's cruelty, but trust that after the first few weeks you'll be dealing just with your sadness without your body putting a magnifying glass on your grief.

If your pregnancy was planned and highly anticipated, the calendar may become your worst enemy. If you know exactly how far along in pregnancy you were when you miscarried, it's hard to resist thinking about how far along you would be now and how your baby would be developing.

It doesn't help if everywhere you turn you see images of babies. Pregnant women. Children. Baby-shower invitations. The littlest things may send you into tears. You might have trouble holding yourself together in public if you see a woman carrying a baby, dragging a preschooler along behind her, and sporting a pregnant belly. You may wonder, "Why can't that be me?" You might hate grocery shopping because when you grab the shopping cart the child seat plops open and the empty space reminds you again of the baby who should be sitting there. You might hate going to work because your coworkers keep inviting you to baby showers, and you just can't handle that right now. Your extended family might criticize you because you don't want to visit your sister-in-law who just gave birth to triplets and can't figure out how she is going to manage.

When a woman's body is going back to a "no longer pregnant" state, she experiences quite a lot of hormonal changes, which tie in with the sadness many feel in the first few weeks. She feels sad because she's had a loss, but the sadness is magnified by hormones. In essence, she's going through postpartum blues. The sadness can feel absolutely scary, as if it's never going to end. But the coming of your period means your body has straightened itself out hormonally. You're going to feel different, as if you own the sadness.

—Kristen Swanson, R.N., Ph.D., F.A.A.N., professor and chair,
Department of Family and Child Nursing,
University of Washington

Whatever you're feeling, it's normal. There's nothing wrong with you. And you're not alone. One study found that about 32 percent of women studied following multiple miscarriages could be classified as clinically depressed, and that 53 percent had troubles with marital adjustment. But you don't have to have had multiple miscarriages to suffer traumatic grief. Another study that looked at women in the week following a first miscarriage found high levels of anxiety (apprehension, tension, uneasiness) in 41 percent of the women and symptoms of clinical depression (depressed mood, feelings of worthlessness and guilt, insomnia) in 22 percent.

If your feelings following your miscarriage are interfering with your ability to function in your daily life and you're concerned that you may have clinical depression, I highly recommend that you seek an experienced counselor who can help you find ways to cope. You're dealing with a terrible loss, and it's okay to need help to get through it. You shouldn't have to face the world alone.

The most important thing to know is that, regardless of what happens, you won't feel this bad forever. If you're in those first few horrible days after a loss and someone has just given you this book, you might feel as if your pain will never end. You have to give yourself time. Trust me: You will go on, somehow. I'd be lying if I said your pain would go away completely, but you will get to a point at which you can bear it.

I feel traumatized by the miscarriage. I feel sad that I am not pregnant anymore. I am sad for my husband. Although it is not rational, I feel betrayed by my body. I feel more irritable now, and I need to have more time to myself.

—ALYSON

After about a month following each miscarriage, I began to feel better and to scrape up the strength and courage to try all over again in all aspects of my life. But the hurt goes on like the river Styx—always running deep. It never leaves you, but I developed a new strength and an acceptance that life does go on, while sad things happen all the time.

—LISA

I felt lost. I felt numb. I knew I needed to snap out of it but I felt like I was in a hole and I could not get out of it.

—Angela

It changed my whole life, how I saw the world. I told my mother it's like rape. When you hear about someone being raped, you feel terrible for them, but you don't walk around paranoid. But if you yourself were raped, you would never see the world the same way. You would lose your faith and live in fear. It's the same with miscarriage. I am no longer naive.

—Janice

Once the shock wore off, and I realized I'd lost my baby, it took me several months to begin to feel normal again. I had difficulty getting up in the morning, getting to work on time, and working. I spent a lot of time online at pregnancy-loss message boards. I was let go from a job four months after the loss, and I feel my depression played a part in that.

—Sherry

Don't fear that if you seem to need a tremendous amount of energy just to get through the day that you're abnormal in any way. This is totally normal. And if you and your partner are handling the loss differently, that's normal, too, and is another part of miscarriage you may need help coping with.

Your Relationship with Your Partner

Many couples find themselves facing relationship conflicts in the aftermath of a miscarriage, especially if they don't feel the same about the loss. Divides frequently happen when a woman is devastated by a loss but her male partner seems to recover quickly. Typically, the woman is wracked with grief and does not understand why her partner seems to resume the functions of day-to-day life more easily. She begins to resent her partner for not caring that they lost the baby. Her partner, meanwhile, is feeling sad about the loss but not overwhelmed by it, and he can't understand why she seems to have gone off the deep end. The partner wants to support her but looks forward to when life will return to normal.

Occasionally this strain leads to the end of a couple's relationship. The woman is left unexpectedly single, grieving the loss of both her partner and her baby.

In the first few days after a miscarriage, men are like their spouses—very sad about losing a pregnancy and their baby. They may even have a similar awareness of the baby as "my child." The woman gets even deeper into this awareness that she's lost the baby. Seventy-five percent of women who miscarry would tell you they lost a baby. With men the loss is just not quite as real. What ends up happening next for the man is more a sense of losing her. She is still grieving. He's gone through the initial sad days, and now he wants to get close again and go back to being pretty joyful. He may be moving on, callous, and he will judge her as carrying on a little too much when it's time to move on.

—Kristen Swanson, R.N., Ph.D., F.A.A.N.

If you find your relationship strained after your loss, it's important to remember that this is one of the many areas in which people are different. More often than not, grief after miscarriage just doesn't hit both halves of a couple evenly.

Studies that have examined couples' grieving patterns show that men's grief differs from women's but that in most cases men do grieve pregnancy loss. A study by German researchers followed 56 couples after their miscarriages. The study found that, contrary to expectations, the male partners grieved, but their grief was not as intense as the women's, and the men felt less need to talk about it. This difference was often a source of tension between the partners.

> I put a bit of a barrier between us because I felt the grief so intensely and wanted to be alone with my pain. Eventually I started opening up, and this actually made us closer.
>
> —Gloria

He was sympathetic and obviously upset that I was upset, but not upset about the actual miscarriage at all. He just didn't understand. The closest he came to understanding was when I broke down in the parking lot of the clinic and told him that although I didn't want him to feel the pain I felt, I also did want him to feel the pain so he could understand it. He asked what it was like, and I said, "Imagine losing someone very precious to you whom you love and cherish." I told him I had been thinking that with all this stress maybe we should separate. He cried at the thought of losing me, and I felt terrible and apologized. Even though I felt horrible and dirty and guilty for doing that, it helped that he understood a little better.

—GEORGIA

He tried so hard to be supportive, but it was so clear (and he admits) that he didn't understand. He didn't feel the loss and still doesn't. I was so happy when at eight weeks into this pregnancy he actually talked about our new baby as a future child. I think this one is real to him, now that he's seen it on an ultrasound. I wish the other one were real to him, too.

—BARBARA

He was supportive and upset, but admittedly not as devastated as I was. It's different for men, I think. They don't have the connection with the baby. I know he felt very helpless because he couldn't fix this problem.

—SOFIA

I think it is important to talk to your partner about things other than reproduction in the time following a loss, or while trying to conceive again. Sometimes it is a struggle, but we have days where we agree to not think about reproduction, and this helps a lot.

—MICHELLE

After our last pregnancy loss, there were times that I thought our marriage would not survive. We argued quite a bit, but in the end we are still together.

—ZOE

I sometimes feel that was really my last chance to have another child with my partner. Things are so different between us now. I couldn't imagine having sex with him again, let alone a baby.

—CANDICE

My partner behaved like an absolute ass throughout the rollercoaster period when I didn't know whether or not I would miscarry. He said, "There's nothing I can do," and went to the pub. And when I actually miscarried he couldn't look at me. But this behavior was completely out of character for him, so I knew he was really affected by the news.

—ALICIA

It might take effort on the part of both of you to keep your relationship healthy following a loss. Following is advice from my husband, first for you and then for your mate.

TIPS FOR WOMEN ABOUT MEN, AND FOR MEN ABOUT WOMEN, FOLLOWING A MISCARRIAGE
(by Matt Danielsson)

Understanding the Man's Reaction

There's a good chance your partner will develop a sudden urge to start a home-improvement project or dive headfirst into a pile of new work at the office just when you need him the most. You need a shoulder to cry on, someone to listen to your feelings and thoughts, and, most important, you need to get a handle on how the miscarriage is going to affect your relationship, now and in the years ahead.

So of course this is the perfect time for him to attack the problem of new kitchen countertops with a vengeance.

This is not a sign of indifference, and it is most likely not a threat to your relationship. As far as he's concerned, he's dealing with his grief in the only way he knows how: by keeping his hands busy and letting things work themselves out.

To understand why men react this way, you have to realize that most men are rather simple creatures. Give most men a steak and a beer, and they are happy. Turn off the game and ask him to vacuum, and he is unhappy. In terms of emotional complexity, most women are precision Swiss watches, whereas most men are sundials.

When something as big as a miscarriage happens, imagine an emotional overflow on the scale of five gallons of water being poured from a bucket into a drinking glass. Now, women can handle this kind of overflow by talking with friends for hours, crying, eating ice cream, drinking wine, crying some more, and so on until some semblance of balance is regained.

A guy, on the other hand, tends to be uncomfortable crying and hugging his buddies, and he may lack the verbal tools to talk things out. Bear in mind, little boys are told not to cry and to "walk it off" with clenched jaws when something hurts. This conditioning tends to stick. So, instead of talking, a guy gets the urge to do something when misfortune strikes. He may not even be aware of his underlying grief; all he knows is that he has to get started on those countertops right now!

But while he's trying to focus on the exact measurements of the granite slabs, his wife keeps interrupting him every two minutes.

"Don't you have feelings about this? Don't you even care?" she demands to know.

"Sure I do. I think it's terrible."

"Yes, but shouldn't we talk about it?"

"We just did!" he says with a vague feeling of unease, knowing on some deep level that he is as in over his head as a dog trying to comprehend advanced calculus.

Don't try to force him to talk. Frustrating as this situation may be, pushing him to "open up" or "talk about his feelings" when he's upset may have the opposite effect. Give him the space he needs, and he'll be back to his normal self by your side soon enough.

Understanding the Woman's Reaction

It can be hard to watch someone you love go through a miscarriage. What you need to know is that, for your partner, the loss wasn't merely a physical experience, and the baby was more than just an idea. Your partner may feel as if the loss took a part of her away and violated her as a woman. Her baby, who was dependent on her for safekeeping, was ripped from her body in a way that she couldn't control. She may feel that she failed as a mother because she wasn't able to protect the baby, even though she may know that the miscarriage was not her fault. Reason has nothing to do with these feelings of self-blame. Because this happened in her womb, the core of her womanhood, if you will, and she wasn't able to control it, the miscarriage might feel to her like a kind of psychological rape. The severity of the reaction varies from person to person, but for many women, miscarriage is hard to put behind them. The loss stays with a woman, sometimes for a very long time.

Your partner needs to know that you are there for her. Be willing to listen when she wants to talk. Try to let her know how you're feeling, too, even if your feelings aren't as intense as hers. If you don't appear to grieve, she may think this means you don't care that you lost the baby. Let her know that you do care. The more you are able to share your feelings with your partner, the quicker things will probably get back to normal in your lives. A study by researchers at the University of Washington found that couples who shared their feelings with each other after pregnancy losses were more likely to have an improved interpersonal relationship and to return to a normal (or better than normal) sexual relationship than were couples who did not share their feelings.

For more tips for guys on coping with miscarriage, see chapter 8.

It is quite important for a couple to learn how each of them deals with stress. Often, partners deal with stress differently, and this can lead to feelings of isolation and eventual disappointment and anger with each other. For example, some people may deal with stress by gathering information and talking about the information and their feelings. Other people may cope with stress by distancing themselves from the problem and withdrawing.

It is very helpful for a couple to see a therapist with a specialty in reproductive medicine soon after a miscarriage, for a consultation (not necessarily ongoing treatment) to help them cope with this major life stressor and to elucidate what each of them needs from the other. An initial consultation can help a couple work together from the outset and prevent isolation. Sometimes just learning what the normative emotional experience is for couples is quite helpful. Prevention is the best cure.

It is very important for the couple to let one another know what they need (in as exact a way as possible) and not to assume the other will automatically know ("I need you to ask me how I feel before you check the mail").

It is important to share fears and worries. It is not uncommon for people to feel that their partners will abandon them or are disappointed in them or blame them. It is important to communicate these feelings so that they don't turn into firm beliefs about the marriage.

Going to doctor appointments together is helpful. It is important to do things that convey to each other that miscarriage is about the couple and family and is not a personal event.

—MADELINE LICKER FEINGOLD, PH.D.

Both of you need to know that you are each other's rock. You are in this together, and you are each other's best companion in facing what you've been through because you've been through it together. Make your relationship with your partner your first priority, and do everything you can to be available for one another.

When You Don't Have a Partner

If you are not in a committed relationship and have experienced a pregnancy loss, you may be feeling particularly lonely—especially with all this discussion of relying on a partner for support. You are more likely to be told that "it was for the best," and your medical practitioner may take less seriously any desire you have for tests and trying again. You need support as much as anyone else who has lost a pregnancy. If you are not able to lean on friends and family, I strongly advise finding a support group, if not in person, then online.

Facing the World

Insensitive comments are the bane of everyone who's experienced miscarriage. You may feel at times as if everyone in your life has something insensitive to say to you about your loss.

When people offer such comments, remember that they probably aren't trying to be hurtful. They may honestly want to help. After all, it can be hard to know what to say to someone who has just miscarried, especially for people who have no personal experience with pregnancy loss.

People who have experienced other losses, such as stillbirth or the death of a child, may compare their experiences to yours in a belittling way. They may say things like "Imagine how bad you'd feel if the baby died *after* it was born." Even though you may feel that a later loss would be worse, remember that you have a right to grieve. Don't feel the need to compare your loss to other kinds in an attempt to validate your feelings.

In your search for support, remember that other people can't read your mind, and if they haven't been through miscarriage before they may not be aware of what they can do to best support you through the experience. Don't be afraid to speak up. This applies to your partner, your friends, and even your practitioner. People often don't know what you need unless you tell them.

Remember, too, that miscarriages are very common. You may find a sympathetic friend where you least expect to.

Limit the phone calls. Some people know just the right things to say, but others are cruel without meaning to be. They rub salt into your raw wound. They may imply that the miscarriage was your fault, but of course it wasn't. You can do nothing to prevent an impending miscarriage.

—Cassandra

Friends and family who hadn't had a loss didn't really even acknowledge that I had lost another child. Some never even said they were sorry. It is frustrating when sometimes you want or need to talk about things and they act as if nothing is wrong or nothing ever happened.

—Tammy

Author's Story

Now that I have come out on the other side, when I encounter someone who has had a miscarriage my first inclination is to offer advice. Because I'm a compulsive researcher into all the problems I encounter in my life, my instinct is to talk about what the person should look into, what she should ask her practitioners, what tests might tell if there is a problem that could lead to more miscarriages. I want to reassure her that answers may be within her reach. I want to distill into just a few minutes all the information that I spent months accumulating when I was in the depths of my own despair. After all, when I went through my miscarriages it was really hard to find this kind of information!

But then I have to remind myself that not everyone wants advice and not everyone takes my approach to things. Sometimes the right reaction is just to say, "I'm sorry for your loss." Grief is very personal. What may be condolence to one person may aggravate someone else's pain.

My sister was very supportive, as she had had a stillbirth, and a lot of friends and family members sent cards, called, and brought food over. But by the next week it had all stopped. I have never felt so lonely as I have the past five weeks. They call, but they never ask how I am recovering from the miscarriage; it's as if no one wants to go there. I sometimes sense they feel uncomfortable when I bring it up. And I do bring it up, because our baby Cole was a part of my life and always will be.

—JODY

Having the support of loved ones and a busy job made me switch off my grief during the day. The nights were the hardest.

—SUZANNE

Many of my coworkers have suffered losses but went on to have children, and hearing their stories gave me hope.

—MEGHAN

In most instances of grief, it helps to find people whom you can lean on. But after a miscarriage you might find that other people cause you even more grief. It's okay if you want to be alone. You shouldn't feel pressured to go to parties and interact with people at social functions if you just aren't feeling up to it. If you're an extrovert, you might take comfort in sharing your loss and feelings with close friends and in being with people. If you're an introvert, though, you might find being around people to be taxing and might take more comfort in being alone. Either way of coping is okay.

If you have to shield yourself from the world to avoid images of babies and children for a while, do it. As you'll see in the comments that follow, you're not alone if you lose your composure every time you see a pregnant woman or baby.

> *My sister found out she was pregnant the week I miscarried. She had a rough pregnancy and complained about everything. I would have given anything just to still be pregnant! One of my best friends got pregnant in her first month of trying to conceive, but she was unhappy that her due date would be in July, the hottest month of the year. Little things like that would set me to crying again.*
>
> —TAMMY

> *I do not attend baby showers, and everyone is very understanding about that. Sometimes just seeing a baby can hurt very deeply. I try to remove myself from any situation that makes me uncomfortable or too sad. I also don't celebrate Mother's Day.*
>
> —SUSIE

> *I would get really mad if I saw a woman smoking and she was pregnant. I just wanted to yell at her and tell her I had just lost a baby and I did everything to make sure it was healthy and she was smoking as if she did not care.*
>
> —KRISTY

> *After my miscarriages, I became another person. I was angry and bitter. I hated all pregnant women and felt that every one of them was less deserving than I was. After I decided to stop treatment and*

pursue adoption, I started being a nice person again. A huge weight was lifted off of me.

—MARINA

The hardest thing for me was seeing my pregnant sister-in-law, who had a baby two months after the miscarriage. Seeing my niece didn't really bother me, but I just could not see my sister-in-law while she was pregnant.

—EMILY

My sister, who has never had a miscarriage, insisted I have a baby shower for her three months after my first miscarriage. I practically cried my way through it.

—PAULA

It is most difficult to face women who had a baby around the time my baby should have been born. Invitations to baby showers are difficult as well. Just shopping for a baby outfit for someone else's baby breaks my heart. I recently attended my sister's baby shower, and I had to leave the room as she was opening her gifts. While I am happy for other women who have the joy of a successful pregnancy, they are a painful reminder that my baby was lost.

—JENNIE

Every time I see a baby or a pregnant woman, I get this awful feeling in my stomach and a lump in my throat, and sometimes I have to fight back tears.

—HEATHER

I try to be happy for people, but when I hear of women having healthy babies while using drugs or people who are abusive to their children I do get bitter. I wonder more and more what's wrong with me, when I'm trying to do everything the right way. I get ads for baby stuff in the mail, and my husband tries to get to them before me so he can throw them away before I see them.

—LAKEESHA

Author's Story

I have a very clear memory of a time, about two weeks after my second and hardest loss, of seeing a happy family walking together: a two-year-old, a baby, and a mother who looked about five months pregnant. Why, I wondered, was she a "fertile Myrtle" when I couldn't even have one child? I wasn't a bad person, was I? How was it that even drug users and alcoholics could carry healthy babies to term but I couldn't even get out of the first trimester? I ate healthfully. I exercised. I took care of myself while pregnant. It just wasn't fair.

Two years later, having conquered the miscarriages, I was walking on a trail near my home with my two-year-old in tow and my belly visibly pregnant. I caught the eye of a woman walking with her partner, and I recognized that look of despair as we briefly made eye contact. She looked away with a steely face and gripped her partner's hand. That was me, once upon a time. I wanted to grab her, give her a hug, and tell her it was going to be okay. I wanted to tell her to keep trying and keep believing that she'd be holding her child someday, too.

Keep in mind that the woman you're so envious of, with the toddler and the newborn baby, might have gone through hell to get them. The baby might be adopted. The mother might have been through six rounds of in vitro fertilization and spent $100,000 before she got her miracle.

The important thing is that the other side of this tunnel looks the same to everyone, no matter what the journey is like. Try to spin your thinking so that seeing babies everywhere you look gives you hope. Odds are that one day you'll be on the other side, too, and, when you are, the women looking at you with envy and sadness won't be able to see all the hard work it will have taken you to get where you are.

When you wake up each morning in the aftermath of your loss, remember that you are one day closer to the end of your struggle with miscarriages. Every day you wake up is a day closer to the day you hold your baby. It may take time, but time passes. On the day you first meet your baby, all of this waiting and pain will be a memory. And it will have been worth it.

I cry every time I see babies and ads for baby things. I have two preg-
nant friends, and I find it hard to be with them. They have been very
supportive, but I am dreading when they start showing and their
babies are born.

—GWEN

I could not watch any TV show, factual or dramatic, in which a
woman gave birth. I would get tearful if I heard of a birth or saw a
newborn or a heavily pregnant woman. I avoided christenings.
Even a diaper ad could make me cry on a bad day.

—CAROLINE

On my first day back to work, a coworker had her three-month-old
grandson at the office "showing him off." That was one of the worst
days of my life.

—TAMMIE

Understanding Grandparents' Grief

Depending on the dynamics of your family, you may face a number of
reactions from your parents and your in-laws following your miscarriage.
They may be completely indifferent to the loss, and they may be among
the people making insensitive comments at every turn. They may be very
concerned about you and how you're feeling. Or they, too, may be grieving for the baby. Remember, the child you were carrying would have been
their grandchild. Particularly if your pregnancy would have resulted in
their first grandchild, they may be going through a loss of expectations.
They may have told their friends about the pregnancy and may be reeling
now after having been giddy with excitement over their grandchild.
Talking with your parents or in-laws about your shared loss may be therapeutic for all of you.

If You Have Other Children

Talking with your children about your miscarriage may be difficult, particularly if they aren't old enough to understand complex issues like birth and death. Very young children might be completely oblivious to what happened, especially if the loss occurred early in pregnancy. But if you miscarried after telling your children that you were going to have a baby, then you need to talk to them about it. It is most important to explain that the miscarriage wasn't their fault or yours. Use appropriate language; you might say, for example, "It was an accident." Check with your children later so they have a chance to share their feelings with you. For more advice, see "Talking to Children about Pregnancy Loss," published by the United Kingdom's Miscarriage Association and available at the association's Web site (see Appendix B).

On a related note, if you have living children you may find that a lot of people assume you won't grieve miscarriages in the same way as someone who doesn't already have kids, and they may tell you that you should be thankful for the children you have. Don't feel that you must minimize your grief because you already have children. It's okay to be both thankful for the children you have and sad about the baby you lost.

> *I have one son, and having him helped me cope. I had a reason to keep on going. Without him I don't think I would be nearly as mentally healthy.*
>
> —Jennifer

> *I got a lot of comments like, "Well, go hug your other children for a while tonight." I am learning what* not *to say to someone who has experienced a miscarriage.*
>
> —Cassandra

> *I feel very lucky to have my children, which does help to cope through a loss, but many people assume that just because you have other kids the miscarriage really didn't matter.*
>
> —Vanessa

I have a five-year-old, and I felt that the only place I could cry was in the shower. My daughter was so sad already that I didn't want her to see the true depth of my grief. I didn't want her to worry that she wasn't enough for me. But having my daughter made the experience easier for me. I think it would have been worse to lose a first baby.

—WENDY

Facing Unsupportive Practitioners

Every part of the miscarriage experience can be taxing. This is true even of your relationship with your practitioner. Many women are dissatisfied with the medical care they receive following a miscarriage. Many physicians rush through appointments, forget that what is perfectly common and clinical to them is devastating to their patients, and ignore that a routine day in which they deal with a couple who have lost a baby may be the worst day in the lives of that couple.

I lost my baby because of low hormone levels. I knew this was a problem, but I couldn't get the nurses to understand the urgency. They would not change my appointment to an earlier date because they felt I was being a typical expectant mom. I wish I had called them every day, three times a day. I'm not a pushy person by nature, but in this instance I wish I had been.

—A. J.

One doctor told me it was my fault, because I went hiking while pregnant.

—TINA

I hated that the doctors kept saying, "Unfortunately, miscarriages happen a lot. It's just nature taking its course." The exams were not as gentle as I needed. I needed someone sensitive to the emotional side of pregnancy. The hospital should have a social worker on staff who attends to pregnant women in the emergency room.

—JODY

Before the losses I always followed my doctor's every word. Afterward, I researched, I asked questions, and sometimes I got the feeling I was irritating her. But she always took the time to talk to me and give her point of view.

—Tammy

My doctor was wonderful; he was very sympathetic. He gave a lot of information and answered all the questions that he could. He even told us that his wife had had a miscarriage last year.

—Melanie

I did not really like my specialist. He was fat-phobic. He told me to come back when I lost 30 pounds.

—Ava

The doctors and nurses in the emergency room were very understanding. They let me hold my little baby, and they took care of my husband by bringing him some coffee and a snack.

—Michelle

My doctor told me that I wasn't far enough along to worry about having a D&C. The very next day, I passed everything on my own. I do wish he had prepared me for what I would see.

—Jana

It took me some time before I found a doctor who was sensitive to my situation. My current doctor had his office staff send me a rose after my last two miscarriages, and has expressed his sympathy for my losses.

—Evelyn

Until you experience any high-stakes medical problem, such as recurrent miscarriage, it can be easy to believe that doctors hold the answers to any and all medical ills. Sadly, this is not the case. Doctors are only human, and they have a limited number of tools at their disposal. Modern medicine hasn't solved all the mysteries of the human body. Doctors can do nothing to stop a miscarriage that has already begun and can rarely do anything about a "threatened" miscarriage in the first trimester. Most of the time, the only treatment they can offer for a miscarriage that's in progress is to monitor the bleeding to make sure the woman doesn't suffer a hemorrhage. Some treatments exist for recurrent miscarriage, as described in chapter 3. But practitioners cannot always find a cause for recurrent miscarriage, the treatments do not always work, and much is still unknown about why miscarriages happen and whether anything can be done to stop them.

So, with all this in mind, try to have realistic expectations for what your practitioner can do for you. You should expect your practitioner to treat you with respect and to give you reassurance. If you're not getting the treatment you want, consider whether finding a new practitioner might be the best course of action. Remember, studies show supportive care to be linked with a lower miscarriage rate. Are you going to be comfortable coming to this practitioner when you're pregnant again? Do you feel that he or she pays adequate attention to your concerns and makes you feel comfortable with the answers? If not, then look around for someone with whom you feel more comfortable. Don't be afraid to call offices and ask to interview doctors. When you find someone you like, set up a preconception appointment. You want to have a supportive practitioner ready to begin seeing you very early along in your next pregnancy.

Of course, your insurance plan may limit whom you can see. In this case, you have a number of options. You can tell your current practitioner how you feel and appeal for more help. Remember that most doctors enter the profession with the goal of helping people. Ask for a little extra time, explain your concerns and why you have them, and be very clear about what you want your practitioner to do for you. For example, if you want to have a blood test done to rule out a cause of miscarriage, and your practitioner doesn't suggest the test, ask for it. If when you get pregnant again you would like the doctor to check for the heartbeat early on, and your practitioner doesn't bring up this possibility, ask. The doctor may not be aware of how concerned you are or may simply not think of suggesting a particular test or treatment. If you're too nervous to share your feelings in person, consider writing a letter. And be prepared to pay up front if the tests you request are not covered by your insurance company.

Memorializing Your Lost Baby

Creating some kind of memorial for your baby might help you cope with the loss. This may sound silly at first, but our own psychological needs are among the reasons we bury our loved ones. If your loss has happened far enough along in pregnancy that you can bury the baby, this may be a good way to find closure for your grief. If your loss was too early for you to have anything to bury, you could still participate in a formal group memorial service (or hold your own service). Some hospitals hold regular group memorial services for babies lost to miscarriage and stillbirth. Check with a local support group to find out if such services are available in your area. (You can find a local support group through a national organization such as Share Pregnancy & Infant Loss Support or RESOLVE: The National Infertility Association; see Appendix B.)

Following are other ways to memorialize your baby.

NAME THE BABY

It can be hard to mourn someone who has no name. Naming your baby (and choosing the sex according to your gut feelings) may help you to feel that your baby's personhood is recognized and may give you a more concrete focus for your grief.

MAKE OR BUY A SPECIAL NECKLACE OR BRACELET

Some mothers find comfort in having a special necklace or bracelet to remember their babies, perhaps with a charm such as an angel or a heart. If you have a very small picture or other small item that reminds you of your baby, you may wish to put it in a locket and wear the locket on a necklace to keep the memory close to your heart. Appendix B lists some online retailers that sell miscarriage-memorial jewelry and other items.

PLANT A TREE

You may find a sort of a catharsis in creating a new life to honor the one that was taken from you. Nurturing a tree from seed can be an amazing experience. Or you might buy a young tree from a nursery. Either way, you can plant the tree in your garden or near your home to create an enduring memorial to your lost baby. You can also make a small donation to one of several environmental organizations to have a tree planted in a protected forest in honor of your baby. Save the Redwoods League (www.savetheredwoods.org), TreeGivers (www.treegivers.com), and American Forests (www.americanforests.org) are a few organizations that offer this service.

WRITE A POEM . . . OR ANYTHING

Are you the type of person who copes with troubles by keeping a journal? Consider writing down your feelings about your loss. You might write a poem dedicated to your baby, or maybe an essay. Or you might write in no particular form but just to get everything that's inside you out on paper. You don't have to share your writing with anyone, but you can if you like. You might even post your piece on one of the many on-line miscarriage memorial Web sites, or create your own miscarriage memorial Web site or blog.

ENVISION YOUR BABY AS A PERSON

Trying to envision a face for your lost child may be helpful, particularly if your loss happened later in pregnancy and you saw your tiny baby—a frightening and heart-rending experience. A mental image of your baby as an older child may help you cope. If you're artistically inclined, consider painting or drawing your vision of your child or finding an existing painting or drawing that matches your mental image of the child.

DONATE TO A CHARITY

Pick any charity that is personally meaningful to you, or consider donating to one that specifically focuses on miscarriage. For example, Share Pregnancy & Infant Loss Support (www.nationalshareoffice.com) is a nonprofit charity that provides counseling after miscarriages and advocates for parents' rights. It is funded by private donations. For a $100 donation, you can have a memorial brick placed in the garden around the Angel of Hope at Share's headquarters in St. Charles, Missouri.

My husband and I drove to the beach, sat by the water, and said our goodbyes. To have my husband open up emotionally was beautiful.

—LESLEY

We had Baby Number Three buried, and being able to visit his grave and sometimes place flowers on it has helped us. Each time I experienced a loss, my husband brought me roses, so I also have a dried rose for each of my three babies, in a small box with the date of the miscarriage on a piece of paper.

—YURIE

I bought a miscarriage-awareness bracelet in pink and blue. I also bought a couple of angel figurines to have in the house. Just having these mementos around helps me to cope.

—EMILY

My husband bought me a ring with the birthstone for the month in which our baby was due. Every time I look at it, I am reminded that I am a mommy and that for a short time I had something precious inside me.

—MICHELLE

I have jewelry with my babies' birthstones on it, and a framed picture of an angel as a tribute to each baby.

—MEGHAN

I have written a poem, and I am planning to buy a glass angel to place by it. I think that this will help me cope and also allow others to remember my baby.

—KIMBERLY

On the anniversary of each loss, my husband and I set off balloons.

—FRANCESCA

I got a tattoo after my first loss. I also wrote letters to my babies. All helped me cope.

—KATHRYN

I planted a white tree that blooms in spring. I lit a candle under the tree, and watched it burn away in the night. I felt peace sitting out among the stars watching the candle burn. This was how I tried to get close to my lost one and connect with the universe to help heal the intense pain of that first week.

—LISA

We bought Christmas ornaments with all our babies' names on them.

—PAULA

We got a stepping-stone for our flower garden. On Tommy's birthday, we are planning to hand out water to walkers at a local park. Water is the symbol of life.

—KAREN

My husband bought me a ring with our baby's name on the outside and little footprints all around. On the inside are the words "It was then that I carried you. . . ." This reminds me that Jordan is in the safest place possible, up in heaven in the arms of Jesus, waiting for me.

—SHERRY

I keep the pictures from the ultrasounds in my pregnancy book, and after one of the miscarriages I even bought an outfit that would have been for the baby I lost.

—SYLVIA

We had him cremated, and the priest is burying him at the memorial garden, where there is a plaque with his name engraved. A few family members will be at the burial—the ones who are supportive. I am hoping this will give us a place to go to when we need it, a beautiful garden.

—JODY

We thought about buying a plant, but we knew that if it died we'd be devastated again. So my partner bought and named a star after our "Angel Pip."

—MORAG

Getting Through the Day

Some days are going to be harder than others. Some days you'll probably feel fine, and other days you'll just want to curl up in a little ball and hide for a while.

Give yourself a break when you need it. If you need to cry, do it. Let yourself feel what you need to feel so that you can get through the experience. Lean on people who make you feel better. If you're religious or have even the slightest spiritual inclinations, you may find comfort in attending religious services and spending time in prayer, either alone or as part of a congregation.

Reading is another activity that you may find helpful. Besides this general book on miscarriage, there are books devoted to couples' heartfelt writings about the experience of miscarriage. Reading such books can be cathartic.

Forgiving Yourself

I'm sure you know that this isn't your fault. Your practitioner has probably told you that, and in your head, you know it wasn't. But in your heart you may not believe it. You may have this nagging voice telling you that the miscarriage happened because of something you did. If you're religious, you might feel that God is punishing you. Even if you're not, it's normal to wonder if you're being punished for some transgression.

I can tell you until the cows come home that your miscarriage isn't your fault, but I know from experience that this may not mean much of anything to you. You have to start telling yourself that it isn't your fault. And you have to believe that it isn't. This is a really hard step to take. Years after my own losses, I'm still not sure I've forgiven my body for not being able to hold onto my babies.

> *I felt I must have done something wrong and was being punished. Before my first miscarriage, I had had a drink (really half a drink) before I knew I was pregnant, and I thought that had something to do with it.*
>
> —MAGDA

> *I felt I should have kept calling doctors until I found someone who would help me.*
>
> —MICHELLE

At times I do blame myself. Who else is there? I wonder if I ate some-thing I shouldn't have or didn't stay in bed long enough every day. I go over all my actions when I was pregnant and analyze what I could have done or didn't do.

—PATRICIA

I feel I have to have a reason so I can fix it. If it's something that I did, it is fixable; I can be in control. When you don't know why, you can't correct the problem.

—MAUREEN

I feel that my stress was a cause, and that without it the baby would have been safe.

—JODY

Finding a Support Group

You don't have to be alone with your grief. If no one in your life has been through a miscarriage, it might help to talk to someone who has. If you need to talk about your feelings with people who understand and your partner is not up for it, or if you are single and do not have a partner to support you at the time of your loss, a support group of some sort may be especially beneficial.

Various pregnancy-loss support groups may meet in your area; to find them, see Appendix B. In the United States, the main support organiza-tion for pregnancy and infant loss is Share Pregnancy & Infant Loss Support. RESOLVE: The National Infertility Association, an organiza-tion formed to help infertile couples, may be especially helpful if you have had trouble conceiving as well as sustaining a pregnancy. If you aren't able to attend meetings, consider checking out some of the online support groups that are also listed in Appendix B. Online forums can give you a free and open place to share your feelings with others who will understand what you are going through.

Attachment can start even before a pregnancy happens; this is one of the reasons why infertility hurts so much. Once a woman is pregnant, she is attached and is a mother. Moms feel it is their responsibility to protect their children, and feel devastated when they can't. Of course, this is irrational guilt when a miscarriage occurs—there is nothing that the mom could have done to prevent it. But feelings are, by definition, irrational.

I think it is helpful for moms to know that feeling guilty is a normal experience, but one they have to combat. Guilt has to do with looking for a reason, a way to understand, a way to assign responsibility. When feelings of self-blame come up, moms have to consciously work to recognize that life can be quite humbling, and that there are times that a mom can do nothing to affect a situation for their children. Miscarriage is one of those times. The self-blame comes from love and attachment and the pain of helplessness.

I think that joining together in a group is often helpful for women who have experienced miscarriage. In listening to someone else's story, it can be easy to recognize that there is no reason for the other person to feel guilty—that she was helpless to do anything to prevent this incredibly sad and devastating event. Sometimes in hearing someone else's story, and in feeling empathy for that person, we can develop empathy for ourselves.

—MADELINE LICKER FEINGOLD, PH.D.

It took several months before I was really able to talk about my feelings, but talking was one of the best tools I found for dealing with all my emotions.

—EMILY

Being able to read online about other people's experiences has really helped to put things in perspective for me.

—YOLANDA

Someone in my online group made bracelets with the birthstones of our babies and sent them to the rest of us.

—Jennifer

I could type things out and clear my head of thoughts that were just going round and round and round with no outlet. I always felt so much better after doing that. When I was ready I moved to the "trying after miscarriage" message board, which was a step up the healing ladder, so to speak.

—Morag

Knowing When to Seek Professional Help

It's normal to be sad and to feel as if you can't go on following a miscarriage, at least for a time. It's normal to feel that the world might end. It's normal to be unable to cope with pictures of babies or pregnant relatives.

But you may reach a point at which it might be wise to seek counseling. If you start to feel even slightly suicidal, seek help immediately. If after a few months you still struggle to get out of bed in the morning and have insomnia, weight fluctuations, inability to concentrate, panic attacks, or other problems that interfere with your daily life, seek help from a psychologist or other mental-health professional. You could be suffering from clinical depression and might benefit from counseling or other assistance. If you and your partner are fighting and not able to get along with one another for months after your loss, it might be wise to seek relationship counseling. Do not be ashamed that you might need help. You have been through a traumatic experience, and adjusting afterward can be very difficult.

I am having panic attacks a lot more often now, especially at night. I think I am not dealing with day-to-day things as well as I used to.

—Michelle

I relive the day I miscarried over and over again, as if my brain is trying to figure it out, trying to cope with the loss. I see images of the operating room, the noises, and the smells. I can't sleep without meds, because my heart just palpitates again and again.

—Jody

I was scared to go out and suffered panic attacks when I did. I felt like staying in bed. I had to get on with life for the sake of my young son, but the miscarriage affected my whole life.

—Isabelle

I was trying to pretend I was fine, when inside I was falling apart. After counseling I realized I was entitled to my feelings, and the second time I handled it much better, because I allowed myself to grieve.

—Jordan

I've had cognitive behavioral therapy, so I'm pretty good at keeping stress from affecting me in the long term. The first two weeks were very bad, but I think that experiencing the pain and grief helped speed my emotional recovery after the bleeding finally stopped.

—Edie

I had to go through therapy to help me cope with the losses. Still, not one day goes by that I don't think about my children and remember seeing their bodies and hearts and faces on the ultrasound.

—Marilyn

If a woman is six weeks post miscarrying and still feels overwhelmed, it would be a good idea for her to check in with an OB or midwife. If she finds approximately three months after miscarriage that she's still overwhelmed with feelings of sadness, counseling would be a very good idea.

—Kristen Swanson, R.N., Ph.D., F.A.A.N.

"Trying Again" as Therapy

For some who have experienced miscarriage, the only therapy is to get pregnant again. In the past, some mental-health professionals advised against trying again too soon after a loss; they believed women should wait until they had fully grieved and come to terms with the previous loss. Like many women, however, you may find that it's cathartic to create new life. Having miscarried may make you more astutely aware of how much you wanted a baby in the first place. A Dutch study found that conceiving again tended to lessen the intensity of couples' grief over a loss.

Maybe you don't want to actively try to get pregnant but won't try to prevent a pregnancy, either. Or maybe you know you're not ready for another pregnancy. That's okay; there is no "right" timing for everyone. See chapter 6 for more on this topic.

Deciding Not to Try Again

Maybe the risk of having another miscarriage is more than you can bear. Or maybe you've been trying to sustain a pregnancy for years, you've tried every treatment available without success, and you've had it with your life being centered on trying to have a baby. Maybe you have living children already and have decided to focus on them instead. Maybe the miscarriage stressed your relationship with your partner enough that you need to focus on fixing that instead of trying to have a child. Whatever your reasons, you're not crazy if you don't want to try again. You have to do what feels right for you in your life.

Maybe you have decided to adopt a child instead of getting pregnant again. After all, parenting is more than just genetics, and there are a lot of children who need loving parents. The adoption process can be tricky and expensive; entire books are dedicated to the process. In Appendix B, I've listed a few Web sites to help you get started in learning whether adoption may be the right route for you.

You may feel an intense loss when you make the decision to stop trying to get pregnant, especially if part of your plan is to actively prevent pregnancy. I suggest you seek counseling if you're not at peace with your decision.

It is very normal (and necessary) to go through a period of grief and mourning after suffering a miscarriage, and this grief and mourning lasts different amounts of time for different people. It can take from weeks to months. Only after sufficient time can one be ready to make a decision about what to do next.

For some, grief and mourning can turn into a clinical depression, and if one is clinically depressed it is difficult to make good decisions for oneself. If mourning lasts more than six months, it may be a good idea to see a therapist (one familiar with issues of reproductive medicine) so that one can be assessed (and treated, if appropriate) for depression. Some signs of clinical depression are depressed mood most of the day and nearly every day, diminished interest in activities, significant weight loss or gain, insomnia or hypersomnia, psychomotor retardation or agitation, loss of energy, feelings of worthlessness or inappropriate guilt, and difficulty thinking or concentrating. If a woman is depressed, I would suggest she treat the depression before making any big decisions.

If a woman is not clinically depressed, but is not feeling resolute about her decision to not try again, I would recommend that, with her partner, she see a therapist who specializes in issues related to reproductive medicine. The goal would be to talk about the effect of the miscarriage on the couple's current decision making and to insure that their decision is based on what is right for them at this point in time rather than on their fears of what may happen. Decisions made out of fear may lead to regret.

It is important for couples to know that there is no right or wrong answer for what they should do—that answer lies within themselves. Sometimes they may need a professional to help them find the right answer for themselves.

—Madeline Licker Feingold, Ph.D.

Author's Story

*W*hen I was feeling the most depressed after my miscarriages, I would think of a calendar. At some day in the future was my baby's birthday. Each day I managed to get out of bed in the morning, I could cross off another day until I'd meet my baby. Whether this would happen in nine months, with a successful pregnancy just around the corner, or after several more years of struggle, I didn't know, but every day was a day closer to when I'd be a mom. And I knew that, even though these times were hard, someday I'd look back on them and feel glad I'd never given up.

Grieve. Don't assume that the loss is not a big deal.

—ROBIN

Lean on your partner.

—PAULA

Keeping a journal is a good way to get your feelings off your chest without feeling like you're bothering others with depressing thoughts.

—CYNTHIA

As hard as it is, be gentle with people who make insensitive comments. They probably mean well.

—JENNIFER

No one wants to be a member of the miscarriage club, but other members are the only people who really understand what you're going through.

—PAULA

You always will wonder what could have been.

—WENDY

If you need to talk with someone, then find the time. Keeping all of your feelings inside will only make it hurt more.

—JANA

Take the time to grieve. Even if you were only four weeks along and had just found out you were pregnant, it was still your baby, and you still feel the loss both physically and mentally.

—TINA

Let other people know that you lost a baby, a precious baby. You never had the chance to hold or see your baby, and you need to be comforted just like anyone who has lost a loved one.

—HEATHER

Be selfish, and don't feel guilty about taking time off to do whatever you feel helps you, even if it's having a really good cry.

—BONNIE

Take some time to think about what is great in your life outside of having children.

— MICHELLE

Try to start making other plans for the near future, even if they are small, to replace the plans you had ripped away from you.

—RACHEL

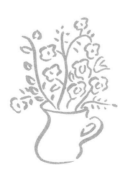

CHAPTER 6

Trying Again

> *We know that another baby will not replace the one we lost—but we want children so badly.*
>
> —DELANEY

IF YOU'RE AT ALL LIKE I WAS AFTER MY LOSSES, you probably view the idea of trying again with a mixture of eagerness and apprehension. You want a baby more than anything, but you naturally fear having your heart ripped to shreds again. You've lost your innocence about pregnancy, and you long for simpler days, when you knew the instant you saw the second line on the pregnancy test that you could start planning your gift registry because a baby would be coming in nine months.

With your innocence gone, you may lean in either of two directions. You may fear trying to conceive to the point that you're practically ready to call an adoption agency. If you feel this way, you're not alone. Miscarriage is this hard on a lot of people. Or you may have become almost obsessed with the idea of getting pregnant again. You may have started thinking of your life in two-week chunks, between the time to ovulate and the time to take a pregnancy test.

When Can I Try Again?

If you want to try again right away, you may be confused by what you hear from your practitioner. No hard and fast rule exists as to the best time to try after a loss; three different physicians trained in different places and at different times may give you three different answers. But generally there isn't a medical reason to wait for most people. One small study looked at medical records and found no increase in the miscarriage rate for those who conceived immediately after a miscarriage versus those who waited. Here are some of the various answers you may hear.

They never said why, but they said three months. Not three cycles, but months.

—JANA

He said to wait for two cycles, because if I got pregnant before then there would be a 10 percent increase in the chance that I would miscarry again.

—LILY

She said that "statistically" it was better to wait at least three months, but she also said that she had had patients who got pregnant two weeks after miscarrying and had uneventful, healthy pregnancies.

—CASSANDRA

He said to wait at least two cycles for physical and emotional recovery. But he also said that no one could tell us when we were emotionally ready; that was our decision, because there isn't a set time to recover from a loss like this.

—JACQUELINE

THREE MONTHS AFTER YOUR MISCARRIAGE

This is the traditional answer. Before the age of high-definition ultrasound, a three-month wait was advised because pregnancy was dated from the last menstrual period, and sometimes three months were needed to reestablish the normal menstrual cycle. But very little scientific evidence supports this long a wait as a medical necessity. Besides, today doctors can date a pregnancy more accurately with an early ultrasound than with the date of the last menstrual period. Yet it's still common to be advised to wait three months before trying again.

In some cases, it may make sense to wait for a few months after a loss. If the pregnancy was further along, especially if your loss was in the second trimester, it could be wise to give your body more time to heal. If you have not been taking prenatal vitamins, a wait could be necessary to replenish the nutrients in your body.

I f you have not been taking prenatal vitamins or other multi-vitamins for the past three months, you should put off getting pregnant until you have been taking them consistently for three months, to decrease the risk of birth defects with the next pregnancy.

—PATRICIA ROBERTSON, M.D.

AFTER YOUR FIRST NORMAL PERIOD

The reasoning behind this is, again, that it is easier to date a pregnancy with a last menstrual period as a reference. Having a normal period also lets you know that hCG (a pregnancy hormone; see page 9) has left your system completely and your body has returned to its prepregnant state. But this common recommendation yet again advises a wait that hasn't been proven to be medically necessary.

RIGHT AWAY, IF YOU FEEL READY

Many physicians these days agree that most women have no medical reason at all to wait before trying to get pregnant again. According to these doctors, once the miscarriage bleeding ceases and the hCG levels have dropped, it's fine for a woman to resume trying. To rule out the remote chance of late miscarriage complications, such as from retained tissue in the uterus, a good practice is to make sure that you test negative on a home pregnancy test before you resume trying.

It is best to ask your practitioner how long you should wait before getting pregnant again. If he or she gives you an answer you don't like, ask for an explanation. Your practitioner could be giving you a "by the book" answer based on the old rationale about dating the next pregnancy, or a recommendation based on your specific medical circumstances. It could be, for example, that tests performed while you were treated for your miscarriage uncovered a problem, like hypertension or anemia, that should be controlled before you get pregnant again. If there are no specific medical reasons for you to wait, however, you might ask if your practitioner feels there is any major risk in trying again right away. If not, it's up to you to decide when you are ready.

Women can try again as soon as the beta hCG is back down to zero and we know they don't have gestational trophoblastic disease (see page 23).

—Mark P. Leondires, M.D., F.A.C.O.G.

Are You Ready to Try Again?

Assuming you have no medical reason to put off trying to conceive again, the most important factor in your decision is how you feel. You need to feel ready to handle pregnancy and to accept the possibility of another loss.

For some women, and sometimes for their partners, actively trying to conceive can be therapeutic; it can help greatly in the process of coping with pregnancy loss. Instead of letting the calendar remind you of how pregnant you ought to be, you can instead use it to track your ovulation and time your pregnancy tests. Wanting to resume trying right away is perfectly normal.

If you don't want to try again right away, that's okay, too. You may be too shaken from the loss to even contemplate another pregnancy. A woman may be deeply fearful of having another miscarriage, and her partner may be unwilling to risk watching her go through one again. You may choose to wait so that you can pursue testing to check for a treatable cause of your miscarriage, or you might just need time to cope with your feelings about what happened. This, too, is normal.

Don't let anyone pressure you into trying to get pregnant again until you feel ready. There is no single way that you should feel after a loss. Take your time grieve the lost baby and get your spirits back up.

One challenge you may face in deciding when to try again involves your relationship with your partner. I think that sometimes my husband wished that we would take a break from trying to conceive, or at least from actively trying. A lot of the time I was so focused on my grief over the losses that I almost forgot about him. He didn't seem to grieve the miscarriages in the same way, and I almost wonder if the hardest part for him might have been the way we lost each other to my obsession with trying to conceive. Nearly everything I talked about concerned getting pregnant. We were never intimate for fun anymore; it was all about "doing it" on the right days to make a baby. My husband was so supportive of me that it was easy to forget that he had feelings and needs of his own.

In deciding when to try again, it might help for you to sit down and have a heart-to-heart talk with your partner at a time when both of you are fully relaxed. Be open about your feelings, and try to understand your partner's concerns. If your partner has reservations about trying again, find out exactly why. Maybe he's tired of constantly thinking about conception and wants to focus on your relationship as a couple (or on your existing child or children, if you have any), or perhaps he's concerned about your emotional health and doesn't want to see you crushed again if you should experience another loss. If you want to try to conceive again right away, validate your partner's feelings, and try to find a way to resolve his concerns.

If you're the partner of a woman who has miscarried, understand that trying to get pregnant again may be therapeutic for her. If you have concerns, please put them out in the open. Just as you cannot read her mind, she cannot read yours. If she understands why you are concerned, the two of you can work through it together.

> *We are ready to try again. The wait has been good. It gave me time to grieve and get back to my life.*
>
> —NATALIA

I wanted to try again right away, because I felt I wasn't doing any-thing to change the situation unless we were trying. My husband said he'd do whatever I wanted, whenever I was ready.

—MEGHAN

I needed to wait that month, but I was desperate to start trying at the end of it.

—TESS

The doctor said I had to wait two months to emotionally heal, as if she could know my emotional healing process. I felt my doctor should have stuck with treating my physical body. I was ready to start trying to conceive again immediately.

—WENDY

I was scared of having another loss but I wanted a baby so badly I just picked up and did all the obsessive charts and tests all over again.

—TAMMY

I was ready to try again right away, and so was my husband. We didn't feel we were trying to replace the babies we lost. We just wanted to have a baby we could hold and love.

—HANNAH

Both my husband and I want me to get pregnant again, but neither of us feels that we need this to happen right away. I do not want to rush; I want to give my body and my soul enough time to heal.

—ALYSON

After each miscarriage I go through a phase of not wanting to ever get pregnant again. After a little while I decide that I want a baby, and I convince myself to try again. My husband supports me in any decision, but I think he is scared of my getting pregnant.

—HEATHER

I want to wait for a while. I am terrified of this happening again, and I want to be as healthy as possible. My husband feels the same way I do.

—CASSANDRA

When You Have to Wait

Having to wait before trying to get pregnant, for medical or other reasons, can be excruciating. You might wake up every morning thinking about getting pregnant, spend your whole day at work daydreaming about it, and go to bed at night thinking about it. Having to use birth control when you want a baby can be especially frustrating.

Even after you start trying to conceive, you face difficult waits. There is the wait to ovulate, the wait to find out whether you're pregnant again, the wait to see if the baby has a heartbeat. Probably the best way to pass the time is to take care of yourself. Focus on reducing stress and keeping yourself as healthy as possible. If there is any aspect of your life other than miscarriage that causes you stress, think about how you can reduce that stress. Consider whether any of the suggestions in chapter 5 might enhance the quality of your life and make you happier with yourself. If you're not taking a prenatal vitamin and mineral supplement, consider doing so (see page 158). You could also ask your practitioner to run blood tests for common nutritional deficiencies (particularly folate and, if you are vegetarian, vitamin B_{12}) and anemia. Addressing nutritional and other health concerns may help you to feel that you're doing something constructive—that you're preparing for your baby while you wait to conceive.

To pass the time, consider taking up a new hobby. Perhaps there is something that you've always wanted to try but never got around to starting. Take an art class, or learn to play a musical instrument. If you already have kids, make your new interest a family activity. The key is to pick something that interests you enough to keep you from thinking about pregnancy all the time.

I find the waiting very difficult. I am passing the time by trying to keep busy and reading books about pregnancy after miscarriage.

—ANNA

I worked a lot, read a lot, and cried a lot. I sank into a deep depression while I watched three "eggs" go by. My husband and I took a vacation, which helped a bit, but even in Las Vegas, I found myself thinking of my lost child and crying.

—MEGHAN

Waiting was hard. I did acupuncture, exercised, and tried to focus on getting ready to try to conceive again.

—WENDY

I had to get myself in check before I felt I could try again. I learned some new crafts and busied myself in the meantime.

—DENA

Hiking and mountain biking are great ways to keep your mind off things.

—MICHELLE

I passed the time one day at a time, counting each day until ovulation and when I could take a pregnancy test.

—BETSY

I counted down every day until we could start trying again.

—EMILY

Choosing a Good Prenatal Vitamin-and-Mineral Supplement

Although a balanced diet should provide most of the nutrients you need, the March of Dimes, an organization that focuses on preventing birth defects and prematurity, recommends that all women of childbearing age take a daily multivitamin supplement that includes 400 micrograms of folic acid, or folate. Taking a multivitamin might be especially helpful for a woman who has had a miscarriage and is planning to conceive again.

When choosing a prenatal vitamin supplement, remember that the nutritional supplement industry isn't highly regulated, and that not all prenatal multivitamins are equal. For example, some contain levels of vitamin A that are higher than is considered safe. High doses of iron and selenium can also be toxic to a developing baby. The March of Dimes recommends choosing a multivitamin that contains no more than 100 percent of the DV (daily value, or the amount that a person should consume every day, according to the U.S. Food and Drug Administration) for each vitamin and mineral. Check with your practitioner before supplementing any nutrient beyond 100 percent of the DV.

You may also want to check whether the supplement you are considering has been tested in a laboratory for solubility. Before the nutrients in a tablet or capsule can be absorbed into the bloodstream, they must disintegrate and dissolve in your digestive system. A 1997 study that examined nine prenatal prescription multivitamin products found that only three of those nine met U.S. Pharmacopeia (USP) standards for the release of folic acid into solution. Most of the others missed the standards by a wide margin; two released only 25 percent of the stated value. Some multivitamin brands have been found to contain lead, and many over-the-counter products have never been tested for either safety or the extent to which the nutrients are released.

Choosing capsules that are filled with powder may be wise, because your stomach acid will dissolve the capsules quickly, and the powder will not need to disintegrate before dissolving. A tablet, in contrast, may pass entirely through your digestive system before being fully dissolved.

To find out which vitamins have been tested by the USP and verified to meet USP standards for purity, solubility, and nutrient quality, visit the USP's Web site (www.usp.org/USPVerified), or look for the "USP Verified" seal on product labels. Remember, however, that lacking USP verification does not mean that a supplement is of poor quality; it just means the manufacturer hasn't had it tested by USP. (An independent lab that also tests supplements and issues a seal of approval is ConsumerLab.com.)

An oft-cited method of testing a supplement's solubility is to place the tablet or capsule in a cup of vinegar (particular instructions vary; ConsumerLab.com suggests heating the vinegar to lukewarm and stirring). If the tablet or capsule does not dissolve in 30 to 45 minutes, then odds are it won't dissolve in your stomach, either.

A Healthy Diet for Trying to Conceive

You hear everywhere that, as long as you maintain a balanced diet, you don't need to change your eating habits. But is your diet truly well balanced? The easy availability of highly processed foods and, especially, junk foods (such as chips and candy), combined with a high-stress lifestyle, can make it difficult to pay a lot of attention to nutrition. I wish I could tell you to discuss this matter with your doctor, but most physicians receive little training in nutrition, and, frankly, the effects of nutrients on the body aren't very well understood in the first place. It cannot hurt to request some tests for nutrient deficiency (such as anemia or folate deficiency) and overall mineral balances within your body, and then to take those results to a dietitian or certified nutritionist and ask what changes you can make to best improve your nutrient status and health. Some insurance plans cover the cost of nutritional counseling. Not only will following any recommended dietary changes boost your odds of a successful pregnancy, but it could improve your mood, energy level, and general health.

Boosting Conception Odds

Conceiving may not be a problem for you; maybe you just have a problem staying pregnant. If you do have trouble conceiving, though, you will want to read this brief overview of how to get pregnant as quickly as possible.

Most women release an egg, or ovulate, roughly two weeks after the onset of the menstrual period. (If your cycles are typically very long, then it's more accurate to figure that you ovulate about two weeks *before* the onset of your menstrual period—on day 21, for example, if your cycles are typically 35 days in length.) Sperm survive in a woman's body for up to five days, and an unfertilized egg can be fertilized for approximately 24 hours following its release from the ovary. So, you're fertile for roughly one week of each cycle. Unless you have very regular cycles, however, it's hard to predict exactly when this fertile week begins.

The most important thing (unless you are attempting to conceive through assisted reproductive therapy) is to have sex at least two to three times a week, to assure the presence in your tubes of sperm that are ready to fertilize the egg. For most people, this is probably good enough. For better odds, though, you can try one or more of the following tactics.

BASAL BODY TEMPERATURE CHARTING

Temperature charting is a fascinating subject. The theory is that your body's core temperature stays fairly stable for the first half of your cycle; then it goes up as much as 1 degree following ovulation and stays elevated until the day before your menstrual period (or, if you have conceived, remains elevated for a longer period of time). Tracking your body temperature over time can help you to pinpoint your usual ovulation date. Couples use temperature charting to prevent as well as to achieve pregnancy.

Temperature charting is the least messy of all the cycle-tracking methods, but it is a little complicated. You have to take your temperature every day first thing in the morning, before you speak or even get out of bed, because your body temperature naturally varies throughout the day and with different activities, and you are trying to detect a pattern of very small fluctuations. Also, temperature charting won't tell you your ovulation date in advance, because your basal body temperature rises only after ovulation. Any movie you may see in which a woman trying to conceive calls out, "My temperature's perfect," is misleading. You can have individual spikes throughout your cycle for one reason or another; it is the consistent elevation that will confirm that you have ovulated. When your temperature has been elevated for three days in a row, you know that you have most likely ovulated three days before.

If temperature charting doesn't predict ovulation, then why do it? If you have consistent cycles, you will be able to predict ovulation, because after charting your temperature for a couple of months you'll know on which day of your cycle you usually ovulate. Practitioners often assume that women ovulate on day 14, but not everyone has a 28-day cycle, and although ovulation normally happens two weeks before the onset of the menstrual period this can vary by a day or two. You might actually ovulate on day 13 or 15, or, if you have longer cycles, day 21 or 22. Charting might help you find *your* usual ovulation date.

Temperature charts can also provide your physician with information about your cycles in the event that they are abnormal. If your temperature rises and falls randomly and you never see a consistent elevation, or if you have fewer than 12 days of temperature elevation between your ovulation date and your menstrual period, this could indicate a possible hormonal problem for which you could be tested. Talk with your practitioner if you think that charting might be advisable in diagnosing the cause of your miscarriages.

You will need a basal thermometer for temperature charting; a regular thermometer isn't accurate enough. You can probably find a basal thermometer in the family-planning area of your local drugstore. Chart your temperature either with pen and paper or on the computer. Multiple temperature-charting software programs are available (see Appendix B).

For more information on basal body temperature charting, see Toni Weschler's book *Taking Charge of Your Fertility,* 10th Anniversary Edition (Collins, 2006).

URINE OVULATION PREDICTOR STRIPS

If you don't consistently ovulate on the same day in every cycle, or if you want to be able to identify your ovulation date in advance, ovulation predictor strips are an option for doing this. They work much like pregnancy tests; you pee on them and then check the line. Most ovulation predictor strips detect luteinizing hormone (LH), which spikes immediately prior to ovulation but is usually present in the body at lower levels. If your LH level is spiking, the test line will be as dark as or darker than the control line. You will want to use the strips for several days before you anticipate ovulating (around the midpoint of your cycle, if your cycles tend to be roughly 28 days long) in order to detect the surge. Refer to the instructions that come with the strips you are using for more information.

SALIVA OVULATION PREDICTOR TESTS

If you don't like to pee on strips, you may instead be able use your saliva to try to predict the fertility window of your cycle. With this method, you smear your saliva on a slide, allow the slide to dry, and then examine it under a microscope. Because of the estrogen surge that happens around ovulation, the saliva should dry in a fern-like pattern of crystals during the most fertile time of your cycle. During the rest of the cycle, the saliva should dry in irregular shapes with no particular pattern. In practice, this method may or may not work; some women get fern-like crystals throughout their entire cycle and others never get fern-like crystals.

If you decide to try this method, don't feel you have to buy a special kit. You can get the same results with a microscope from a toy store.

FERTILITY MONITORS

These are the most expensive of fertility prediction devices, but they are said to take out all of the guesswork. They operate by analyzing urine test sticks for levels of LH. You turn on the monitor on the first day of your cycle (that is, on the first day of your period), and then you turn it on every morning thereafter. In the first month the monitor will indicate around day 8 or 9 of your cycle that you should start using test sticks, and over time it will track your cycles and adjust this date accordingly. When it's time to start testing, prepare your sample with your first morning urine according to the kit's instructions, and then insert the stick into the monitor for analysis. The monitor will tell you whether the stick indicates low fertility, high fertility (when your LH level is rising and you will ovulate within a few days), or highest fertility (when your LH level has surged and you are about to ovulate). Fertility monitors can be very helpful if you have unpredictable cycles, but they are not always accurate. I was using a fertility monitor when I got pregnant with my daughter, and the monitor never detected the surge in LH. It gave me high readings starting on about day 9 and continued to ask me to use test sticks for another two weeks after that, even though I had guessed that I had already ovulated (and turned out to be correct).

Despite all these ovulation-prediction systems, if you're having sex every other day or so, as do many couples who are trying to conceive, you really don't need to know exactly which day you ovulate. Knowing exactly when you ovulate won't by itself boost your odds of getting pregnant if you're already having sex regularly. Tracking an exact date may, however, be important if you or your partner travel a lot or if you need to know your exact ovulation date for medical purposes (to receive treatments or testing).

> *I charted my temperature and monitored my cervical fluid, even during the three-month period in which we couldn't try to conceive. I wanted to see if my body was getting back to normal.*
>
> —MEGHAN

> *I think my stress has just transferred from the actual miscarriage to the mission of trying to conceive again!*
>
> —MORAG

Working with Your Practitioner While Trying to Conceive

If you're struggling with infertility or using some type of medical treatment for recurrent miscarriage, you may have to coordinate your efforts to conceive with your medical appointments. This can be a new sort of hassle in your life. Be sure at every appointment with your practitioner that you understand your treatment plan fully. If you don't understand something, ask. Don't be afraid to bother your practitioner in between appointments if there is something you don't understand. The job of doctors is to help their patients, and this includes answering questions by telephone.

A Note on Pregnancy Tests

As you're waiting for your period to arrive (or not) during the two weeks after ovulation, you may find yourself dying to know whether or not you're pregnant. You may spend a small fortune on home pregnancy tests that are supposed to tell you some days before your period is due whether you're pregnant or not. The abundant "early answer" or "early response" pregnancy tests on the market tend to encourage this spending.

Before you shell out all those bucks for tests, consider the matter. The tests can detect extremely low levels of hCG (see page 9), and so they may tell you earlier that you're pregnant. They can't, however, tell you that you're *not* pregnant. Only the appearance of your period will tell you that for sure. Some women don't test positive with any pregnancy test until the day before or the exact day that their menstrual period is due. So, if you test before your period is due, getting a negative result doesn't necessarily mean you're not pregnant. If you start taking early pregnancy tests the week before your period is due, you might find yourself taking four or five tests each month—which can become expensive if you're using store-bought tests, which might cost $10 apiece. If instead you wait until the day your period is due, you will save money without changing the outcome.

Taking early pregnancy tests can be hard on your emotions as well as your pocketbook. If you test four or five times every month without success, you feel crushed three or four times more often than you need to. In testing early you also risk finding out about "biochemical pregnancies," in which the egg is fertilized but does not implant properly, so that you may test positive but your period still begins the day it is due or shortly thereafter. Emotionally, it may be easier not to know about such conceptions.

Unless you have a medical need to detect a pregnancy as early as possible—for example, your practitioner wants you to begin taking progesterone supplements as soon as a pregnancy can be detected—it is probably best to put off testing until your period is due. But I feel silly advising you to use restraint when I never did myself. I tested every day, sometimes twice a day, watching for the second line to show up. If you just can't help yourself from doing this, see Appendix B. You'll find listed there online retailers that offer extremely cheap, highly sensitive tests in bulk packages of 50 to 100. These may allow you to test to your heart's desire without breaking the bank.

Keeping the Faith

It's hard not to let your feelings get the better of you over something as important as your baby. It's scary when you have controlled everything else in your life, but you cannot control whether you get or stay pregnant. You might find yourself wondering if you'll ever be able to get pregnant again, worrying that you'll miscarry again when you do get pregnant, and working yourself into a depression about what the future may hold.

When such feelings strike, try to remind yourself that biology is on your side. Keep in mind that your body was designed to carry a baby. For most people, there is no good reason to believe that nature won't eventually take its course and that you'll be a mom.

CHAPTER 7

Pregnant Again

> *During my fourth pregnancy, which resulted in a healthy, at-term baby boy, I was a train wreck, always nervous.*
>
> —MEGHAN

IF BEING PREGNANT AGAIN TERRIFIES YOU, you're not alone. If even the prospect of being pregnant again terrifies you, again, you're not alone. You have taped back together the pieces of your heart, and you're hoping it's not going to get broken again. But the fact remains: If you want to give birth someday, you have to take the chance that you may miscarry again. I'm sure you've heard it said that being a parent is like having your heart walk around outside your body. Getting pregnant again is just the first of many heart-rending events you're going to experience along your parenting journey.

The Positive Pregnancy Test

It's not unusual to be happy you're pregnant but not ready to commit to feeling like you're going to have a baby.

Many women who are pregnant after a loss say that they have lost their innocence about pregnancy. Now that you know that miscarriages

> Women describe trying to balance the reality that they could have another loss with trying to do the best they can to have a healthy pregnancy. They say that they can't jump into pregnancy with both feet, because they need to remember that this might not work out. They now feel that pregnancy doesn't necessarily equal a baby.
>
> —DENISE CÔTÉ-ARSENAULT, PH.D., R.N.C.,
> UNIVERSITY OF ROCHESTER SCHOOL OF NURSING

don't just happen to other people, it may be hard to allow yourself to become attached to the idea of having a baby. This is very normal, but beware of letting fear stop you from taking in the experience of your pregnancy.

The first thing you'll probably want to do is get some reassurance. Let your practitioner know that you're pregnant following a miscarriage and would feel better if you could come in for an appointment. At the appointment, talk about your concerns. Your practitioner may not understand that just telling you "Everything is probably going to be fine," doesn't stop you from worrying. Ask your practitioner if you could have serial hCG tests to see if your levels are doubling (see page 5). If they are, that's a great sign. You might also ask if you can have an ultrasound scan at six weeks or so to check for a heartbeat. An early ultrasound is especially wise in a pregnancy that follows a loss due to ectopic pregnancy, to rule out a repeat occurrence.

You may wonder when to share the good news with others. You might regret having shouted it from the rooftops last time, then having to tell everyone that you miscarried. A good rule of thumb when you're feeling more cautious is to start by telling only those people whose support you would need if the worst happened. Then, when you start to feel more comfortable later—such as after you see the heartbeat in an ultrasound scan or complete the first trimester—you might share the news with more people.

Seeing the Heartbeat

As mentioned previously, an ultrasound scan showing a visible heartbeat is probably the best reassurance that you can get in early pregnancy following a miscarriage. Usually the heartbeat is visible by six or seven weeks via vaginal ultrasound. If you've had only one miscarriage and are under age 30, you have a 95 to 98 percent chance of a successful pregnancy when the heartbeat is seen at this point in early pregnancy. This statistic may not be reassuring if you saw a heartbeat before your miscarriage, but an early ultrasound is still the first milestone of your current pregnancy.

If you are over age 30 and have miscarried only once, your chance of a successful pregnancy once you see the baby's heartbeat during a six- to seven-week ultrasound scan is 70 to 75 percent.

If you have miscarried repeatedly, your odds of a successful pregnancy at this point are 70 percent. Many practitioners will offer a second ultrasound scan seven to ten days later to any woman who has suffered recurrent miscarriages. If this second exam shows both the heartbeat and normal growth in the baby, your chance of a successful pregnancy rises to 83 to 85 percent.

Please try not to worry about the baby's heart rate. It's normal for the heart rate to be very fast. It's also normal if it isn't so fast. In the past some doctors wondered if heart rates outside the usual range could indicate a problem, but this does not seem to be the case, at least with a single measurement.

After a loss, women are hypervigilant about every sensation and every symptom they have during pregnancy. They try to decide whether each is something to worry about and whether to contact the care provider or to cry or to pray. Once the baby starts moving, they are reassured. But the early weeks are very anxiety-filled.

—DENISE CÔTÉ-ARSENAULT, PH.D., R.N.C.

If You Have Vaginal Bleeding or Spotting

You may find yourself running to the bathroom every 10 minutes to make sure you're not spotting, and examining the toilet paper thoroughly for any sign of a problem. Even some women who have never miscarried do this. If you do see signs of spotting, try not to panic. One large study found that 22 percent of women who had successful births reported having experienced vaginal bleeding at some point during their pregnancies. While following Internet message boards, I learned that some women who have heavy bleeding with clots still go on to have normal pregnancies.

If you do have vaginal bleeding, call your practitioner to have the matter investigated. You may be able to have serial tests to check your hCG levels or an ultrasound scan to try to find the heartbeat. In some way or other, your practitioner should be able to determine whether or not you are miscarrying and alleviate your concern if you are not.

If you're in the first trimester, I suggest you consider avoiding the emergency room unless your bleeding is heavy—that is, unless you are soaking a sanitary pad in less than an hour. You should certainly go to the emergency room if you are having severe pain (because this could indicate an ectopic pregnancy) or if for some other reason you feel your health is in danger, but for most instances of light to moderate vaginal bleeding it is probably best to call your OB-GYN for guidance. The experience of going to the emergency room may be an added stress that you don't need.

Handling Anxiety

If you're worrying nonstop, you have to find some way to relax. I feel like a hypocrite writing this, because I was extremely anxious in my first successful pregnancy following my miscarriages, and when people told me to relax I felt they were implying that I was being silly for feeling as I did about losing my babies. I felt that these people were telling me to bottle up my feelings and toss them away, as if my feelings about the losses weren't worth anything.

People who are telling you to relax may not understand what you're going through and may not recognize the validity of your feelings. It's normal to be afraid. It's normal to go through the first few weeks of pregnancy following a miscarriage thinking of nothing but the possibility of miscarrying again. But stress isn't good for you. You need to find a way to get control of your heart and let your brain take over for a little while. Talking about your fears can help, but only if your listeners are supportive. If you lack supportive people to talk with, look for a support group for women who are pregnant after a loss (see Appendix B).

Support groups provide a safe, caring environment in which women and their partners can express their worries and concerns. They can talk about their babies who have died, and their feelings and thoughts are accepted as normal. This relieves their feelings that they are going crazy and or that they are abnormal. The support groups I studied were very, very helpful. Many participants said they couldn't get through their pregnancies without the support of these groups.

—DENISE CÔTÉ-ARSENAULT, PH.D., R.N.C.

When you feel yourself getting too agitated, sit still and meditate. Think of yourself as sending energy waves to your baby. Picture your baby growing and developing as he should. As you imagine your baby inside you, silently tell him how much you love him. Tell yourself that you're a woman, with a body designed to support a baby. Nature is on your side. Your body can carry a baby. (You don't need to do this to avoid miscarriage, of course, but it may help you relax.)

If you have a supportive practitioner, you may be offered an early ultrasound scan. If not, your practitioner might be willing to check for the baby's heartbeat with a Doppler device at eight or nine weeks. Depending on the position of the placenta and other factors, the heartbeat may become audible anywhere from seven to twelve weeks along in a normal pregnancy. Some doctors refuse to do a Doppler check until after twelve weeks, to avoid causing unnecessary stress on the mother in case the heartbeat isn't audible before that time. If your practitioner does do an

Author's Story

I rented a Doppler device with both of my successful pregnancies, and I found it to be a lifesaver. With my daughter, particularly, I had debilitating anxiety. I was overanalyzing pregnancy symptoms and convincing myself every two or three hours that I was going to have a miscarriage. I couldn't focus on my work, and I couldn't talk to my husband or anyone else except to express my feelings of doom about the pregnancy. I would check every hour for signs of spotting. Without the Doppler, I wouldn't have been able to function at all during the weeks between when my reproductive endocrinologist stopped giving me weekly ultrasound exams and when I started feeling the baby move.

early check—around eight weeks, for example—and you don't hear the heartbeat, *this does not mean that anything is wrong with your pregnancy.*

Some companies offer Doppler devices for rent so parents can listen to their baby's heartbeat at home. These devices cost $400 to $500 to purchase but as little as $89 to rent for an entire pregnancy. Listening to the baby's heartbeat at home might greatly reduce your anxiety by telling you that, yes, your baby is alive and well. Before deciding to rent a Doppler, though, consider that the device may end up causing you stress if at some point you aren't able to find the baby's heartbeat—because the baby has switched positions, for example. Also, remember that the device operates through ultrasound, and that overuse of ultrasound could theoretically affect fetal brain development. If you decide to rent a Doppler, discuss safety precautions with your practitioner. For example, you may want to limit yourself to checking only once every day or two and listening for only a few seconds at a time. An alternative to renting a Doppler is working with a supportive practitioner who is willing to have you come in for a quick scan by an office staff member anytime you feel anxious.

Your anxiety will probably lessen once you pass the point in your pregnancy at which you lost your other baby or babies. In the meantime, celebrate the milestones: seeing the heartbeat in an ultrasound scan, finishing the first trimester, feeling the baby move for the first time, reaching the halfway point in your pregnancy, having a 20-week ultrasound at which the baby appears healthy, and then reaching the point of "viability," usually considered to be around 26 weeks. At this point, your baby would have good odds of survival if he or she were to be born. Once you're in the third trimester, you should feel your baby's movements regularly, and your practitioners may encourage you to call if you don't feel kicks for a lengthy period of time.

Deciding About Prenatal Testing

At some point during your pregnancy, you may be faced with decisions about prenatal testing. Various types of prenatal tests are available, ranging from simple blood tests to somewhat risky procedures such as amniocentesis. Deciding whether to use these tests can present you with quite a dilemma, especially if you know that your losses had chromosomal factors; you may want the information but feel uncomfortable with the risks involved in procedures such as amniocentesis, or you may fear that a false-positive result will only add to your worries unnecessarily. You may encounter pressure from your practitioner to undergo these tests. Remember that you can always refuse testing, because you aren't comfortable with the risks or for any other reason.

ULTRASOUND

Nearly every pregnant woman these days undergoes an ultrasound scan, usually around halfway through the pregnancy, to check the baby's organs and development. If you have had miscarriages, you may have more ultrasound scans to keep tabs on your baby's development. Ultrasound appears to be safe at low sound frequencies, but, as mentioned previously, some research has indicated that too-frequent ultrasound use may cause abnormalities in fetal brain cells. If you have concerns about the safety of ultrasound, you should discuss them with your practitioner. In many cases, ultrasound can provide great reassurance from anxiety and provide important medical information.

CHORIONIC VILLUS SAMPLING (CVS) AND AMNIOCENTESIS

These procedures involve obtaining cells from the baby and then analyzing their chromosomes. CVS is done earlier than amniocentesis—as early as 10 weeks—and is generally reserved for women at higher risk for having babies with serious genetic problems. Although it is more likely than amniocentesis to induce a miscarriage (the risk has been estimated at 1 in 100), CVS is used because many women want to know as early as possible about certain types of genetic problems, especially those that are incompatible with life. The test identifies many genetic disorders, not just Down syndrome.

Amniocentesis is done later than CVS, at 16 weeks. Because it is less risky than CVS, however, amniocentesis is the more common of the two tests. It is most often offered to women over 35, who have higher odds of having babies with chromosomal problems, and to women who have had high results on the blood screening tests.

The question of whether or not to have amniocentesis can be a highly emotional one, which you and your partner should discuss and decide on together. Many women are vehemently opposed to undergoing the procedure, because it does carry a small risk of miscarriage (estimated at no more than 1 in 200) and because they would not voluntarily terminate a pregnancy under any circumstances. Others might decide to get the amniocentesis because they feel they need to know for certain whether or not their babies are fine. Knowing of problems in advance can help families make preparations for dealing with a child with special needs.

NUCHAL TRANSLUCENCY TEST
AND ULTRA-SCREEN

The nuchal translucency test primarily evaluates the risk of having a baby with Down syndrome or trisomy 18 (a fatal chromosomal condition). Many people prefer this test to amniocentesis because it carries no risk of miscarriage. Performed through an ultrasound scan around week 12, the test measures folds in the baby's neck. Certain measurements are correlated with a greater risk of Down syndrome or trisomy 18.

The nuchal translucency measurement is combined with the results of a test of the mother's blood for a more accurate calculation of the risk of Down syndrome or trisomy 18. The manufacturer of this test, called Ultra-Screen, claims that it can detect 91 percent of pregnancies with Down syndrome, with a 5 percent rate of false positives, and 98 percent of trisomy 18 pregnancies, with a 1 percent rate of false positives.

With all prenatal testing of your baby, the decision to accept or refuse the tests is personal. Only you and your partner know the right answer for you.

If It Happens Again

I wish I didn't have to include this section, because I don't want to cause you to worry, although you will anyway. The sad truth is that some people miscarry repeatedly.

If you didn't have any testing done after your last miscarriage, consider asking your practitioner about the possibility of testing now. You may want to have a karyotype of the baby to rule out chromosomal abnormalities and determine whether additional tests are worth doing (see page 34). If you're not already seeing a specialist, find one (see page 193) and initiate an investigation into any medical reasons that you are losing your babies. You should not have to go through another miscarriage "just to see what happens," especially if you have one of the medical conditions that can be easily treated. Refer to chapters 2 and 3 for some possible conditions you might want to check for. Not every doctor is willing to run tests after a second miscarriage, but many are; they wish to save women from unnecessary grief in the event that a treatable cause exists.

Your second miscarriage may be a different emotional experience from your first, especially if you were reassured after the first one that the cause was probably just a random chromosomal anomaly. You may feel completely hopeless, and you may be at greater risk for clinical depression.

Please keep the faith. Seek out others who can support you through this difficult time, and you will get through it.

If It *Doesn't* Happen Again

In my anxiety-ridden pregnancy with my daughter, I kept using home pregnancy tests to see if the line would get darker. It did for the first four days, but then it started getting lighter. I freaked out, but the baby was fine. My breast tenderness suddenly disappeared in the sixth week, just as it had in one of my previous miscarriages. I was pinching my nipples every hour to check for variations in the soreness. Again I was convinced I was miscarrying, but my daughter was fine. My morning sickness vanished entirely overnight in the tenth week, and she was still fine.

I hope you'll be able to relax more in your pregnancy than I could in mine. Following are some general pointers that may help you cope with your feelings.

Do allow yourself to believe that you will have a baby from this pregnancy. Remember, again, that the odds are in your favor. And if you have had more than one miscarriage and ruled out any treatable causes, your odds remain overwhelmingly high for a successful pregnancy, especially with supportive prenatal care.

Don't keep taking pregnancy tests every day to see if the line gets darker. The darkness of the line on a home pregnancy test is not a reliable indicator of a healthy pregnancy. Many things can affect the concentration of hCG in your urine, and the concentration of urinary hCG does not necessarily reflect the levels in your blood. Frequent urine tests will only cause you stress and deplete your bank account.

Don't feel that you have to tell friends and family about the pregnancy until you're ready. This is your body and your pregnancy, and you don't have to share the news before you're comfortable doing so.

Do picture your baby and acknowledge your attachment to her. It's okay to feel cautious at first, but remember that your relationship with your baby doesn't start at delivery. You're a mommy from the start of pregnancy. Your body will nurture your baby for nine months before birth.

Do take time for yourself. If you started a hobby to pass the time while trying to conceive, continue it during the pregnancy to keep your mind off your worries (unless the activity could be dangerous to the baby; check with your practitioner about this). Also consider participating in some type of stress-release activity, such as yoga or meditation (see chapter 5).

Don't spend a lot of time thinking about miscarriage. If you have been participating in pregnancy message boards on the Internet, you may want to avoid them during your first trimester or at least until the point that your anxieties diminish. Every time you see a message about miscarriage, it's going to make you worry.

Don't overanalyze pregnancy symptoms. If you feel nauseated one day and completely fine the next, this doesn't mean you're losing the baby. If your breasts are less sore one day than they were the previous day, this doesn't mean that something is wrong with the pregnancy.

Do see your practitioner for prenatal care. Find a new practitioner if you're not comfortable with the one who has cared for you in the past. Remember that doctors are providing a service to you and not the other way around.

Do allow yourself to enjoy the experience of being pregnant. Ideally, you will reach a point at which you no longer fear that the miscarriage demon is lurking around every corner. Being pregnant is a truly amazing experience. *Don't* let your fear and anxiety keep you from appreciating that.

Don't be surprised if you feel a touch of sadness when your baby is born. Yes, this is a truly wonderful occasion, and seeing your child's face for the first time is like nothing else you'll ever experience. But seeing your baby might also remind you of what you have lost. You may find yourself wondering what your other baby or babies would have looked like, and feel cheated that you never got to see their faces. These feelings are normal. Accept them, and cherish those lost babies in your heart, but *don't* let your longing for them take away from your love for the baby in your arms.

> *Having a baby was the focus of my life for five years. In those five years I had five pregnancies and one live birth. I endured fertility treatments, including IVF, for all five of those years. I'm so glad to be moving on now.*
>
> —Paula

> *Both losses were hard, especially the first. My heart still grieves, even after 23 and 17 years, respectively. But I am overjoyed with the three children I was able to conceive and carry to term successfully.*
>
> —Tammie

Sometimes it's hard to believe you'll ever reach the end of this journey, but odds are that someday you'll be looking back on these times as just a distant memory. If you would like to read some personal stories of other women whose journeys through miscarriage or multiple miscarriages concluded happily with births, please visit this book's Web site (www.aftermiscarriage.com).

Best wishes to you.

A DIFFERENT CHILD

By Pandora Diane MacMillan

A different child,
People notice
There's a special glow around you.

You grow
Surrounded by love,
Never doubting you are wanted;
Only look at the pride and joy
In your mother and father's eyes.

And if sometimes
Between the smiles
There's a trace of tears,
One day
You'll understand.

You'll understand
There was once another child
A different child
Who was in their hopes and dreams.

That child will never outgrow the baby clothes
That child will never keep them up at night
In fact, that child will never be any trouble at all.

Except sometimes, in a silent moment,
When mother and father miss so much
That different child.

May hope and love wrap you warmly
And may you learn the lesson forever
How infinitely precious

How infinitely fragile
Is this life on earth.

One day, as a young man or woman
You may see another mother's tears
Another father's silent grief
Then you, and you alone
Will understand
And offer the greatest comfort.

When all hope seems lost,
You will tell them
With great compassion,
"I know how you feel.
I'm only here
Because my mother tried again."

(For Madoka Marietta Rosalie, from your mother,
remembering with love and not with sadness
our special angel, Rhiannon Roxane Waldron,
February 1, 1997–March 4, 1997)

CHAPTER 8

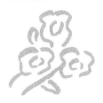

For Dads Only: A Quick Miscarriage Coping Primer

By Matt Danielsson

AUTHOR'S NOTE: In discussions of coping after miscarriage, the fathers often get overlooked. Because I can't interpret the experience from a male perspective, I'm offering here some words of advice from my husband, Matt, based on our experience with three miscarriages. At the end of the chapter you will find comments from women about what their partners did to support them after their losses.

YOU WERE PROBABLY LOOKING FORWARD to the prospect of having a little one perched on your shoulders, laughing and demanding that you run faster or jump higher. With the news of your partner's miscarriage, that vision has been put on hold.

Any doctor will tell you that a miscarriage is nothing to worry about. Miscarriages happen all the time, and odds are the pregnancy will be just fine the next time around. But knowing this doesn't dull the sting. Worse yet, the words sound really hollow if this is the second or third miscarriage you and your partner have been through.

Making matters worse, your partner is probably taking the loss even harder than you are. She may be going through anything from a mild depression to a total meltdown that lasts weeks. Odds are she is looking to you for support. Most guys are conditioned to be stoical, to "tough it out." Feeling pressure to be the rock in the relationship may add to your burden.

Suppressing your emotions isn't healthy. But a lot of talking and "getting in touch with your feelings" may not appeal to you either. You need to find a sensible middle ground, in which you support your partner but have some time to yourself as well. How exactly to find this balance is something only you can determine, but here are some general dos and don'ts.

Do tell your partner that you still love her and that you're there for her. Just say the words and let them sink in. While the fact that you love her may seem obvious to you, sometimes your partner needs to hear it. Consider this the number-one measure you can take to help her to cope and to keep your relationship healthy. It is the biggest favor you can do for both of you, right off the bat.

Don't try to suppress everything you feel. Denial only leads to ulcers. You may feel awkward in the extreme admitting how much the miscarriage affects you, especially at a time when your partner is clearly overwhelmed by her own feelings.

News flash: Women are the experts on emotions! If you want to talk about your feelings, for God's sake, don't hold back. Odds are that your partner will be relieved that you also felt connected to the baby and find reassurance in this. By admitting a little emotional softness, you become all the more of a rock for her. Plus, you may find relief in venting a little.

Do make sure to get plenty of exercise. Nothing relieves tension and clears the mind like some quality time with the punching bag, barbell, or treadmill. Ironically, it's when you're the most stressed that you perceive yourself as having the least time for exercise. For this reason it's a good idea to make commitments to exercise, by booking time with a personal trainer or workout buddy, reserving a racquetball court, and so on. Once you get started exercising regularly, you'll have the same sense of release and refreshment every time.

Don't let yourself become too buried in projects. Keeping your hands busy is a tried-and-true method for staying sane when life throws you a curve ball, so go work on the car or put a coating of weather sealant on the deck. But don't forget your relationship with your partner in the process. If you spend all of Saturday setting bathroom tiles, make sure you do something with her on Sunday.

Do keep a list of "surprise activities" that can be fun for both of you. Your partner will feel down for quite some time. While talking can be therapeutic for men, women, in my experience, need about 10 times more of it. So if your partner needs your attention but you're not feeling up to talking about the miscarriage again, you can save the day by suggesting an activity that you both enjoy. For example, you might say, "Oh, look—a box of chocolate and wine for you, a cold beer for me, and a DVD of that movie we wanted to see!" Or, "Hey, why don't we watch the sunset and have some chowder down at the pier, the way we used to?"

Of course, this won't be appropriate for every occasion. If she is having a particularly hard night, she might feel you're being insensitive by suggesting fun activities. But if she wants to discuss everything that happened for the umpteenth time, an activity that breaks the pattern of your everyday lives may help her cope as well as just talking about the loss.

Good questions partners can ask each other are "How were you attached to the baby?" "What were your dreams in parenting this child?" "How do you mourn, and how is it important for you to mourn the loss of this child?"

—MADELINE LICKER FEINGOLD, PH.D.

Now, you might notice that a lot of this advice involves how to treat your partner. Wasn't this chapter supposed to be about coping yourself, not just keeping *her* happy? Well, in many ways the two are one and the same.

When your partner was pregnant, you learned the cardinal rule that all men learn: Never argue with a pregnant woman. Bite your tongue, and keep her happy. Fail to abide by this rule, and you're opening a can of Just-Add-Brimstone Hell. That's why you put up with being sent out for ice cream at 2:00 A.M., only to come home to a wife seething and sobbing simultaneously because you had the *nerve* to bring her something that's so full of fat when she's already upset about having gained weight (which is normal in any pregnancy)!

The same principle applies in the case of a miscarriage, only more so because of the tragedy underlying the experience. And that's why taking extra measures to support your partner is so important. Being supportive will help both of you avoid conflict and further trouble. Bear in mind that, although for you the miscarriage was a dream ripped to shreds, she may feel like the dream was ripped from her body and washed away in a hormonal storm.

Both of you need a chance to calm down so that you can talk sensibly about what happened, discuss any medical concerns, and determine whether or when to try for another pregnancy. The quickest way to achieve this is to put equal effort into supporting your partner and processing your own grief.

Again, the trick is to find the right balance of "me-time," whether you'll spend it taking an engine apart or crying your eyes out, and support time, during which your primary function is to help your partner get back on an even keel. With this balance, you can't go wrong.

> *My husband was my rock. I don't know how I would have made it without him. I remember only a couple of other friends who helped by listening and not judging me.*
>
> —DARA

> *I got really scared about our relationship after the first loss. Any time he would try to touch me I would literally feel sick. I was scared I would stay that way forever.*
>
> —HILLARY

> *My husband was great. He kept me busy going places and doing things. He also pampered me with hot baths and his cure-all for everything, hot tea.*
>
> —MICHELLE

> *My husband has expressed his sadness in our losing the last two pregnancies. He allows me to cry or talk about the emotional pain of the losses as much as I need to. When he expresses his disappointment and grief over our losses, I feel that I am not suffering alone.*
>
> —ROSA

My husband bought me flowers and helped me a lot by talking about all the things we could do together before trying again. We now have some plans to travel a bit and do other things that we wouldn't have been able to do if I had remained pregnant. He helped me find things to look forward to.

—RACHEL

I was so worried that my husband would blame me or think less of me because I could not protect our baby. So many of my friends' marriages have not survived a miscarriage. But shortly after our first loss he told me that, even if it is always just the two of us, he will consider himself the luckiest man on earth. If our relationship has changed at all, we are closer now.

—MICHELLE

When a man continues to do little things to show he cares, one year post loss, the woman will tell you things are just as good as they used to be. If he talks to her about miscarriage and they share their feelings, the woman will say one year later that they are closer than ever, and that sexually things are at least as good as they used to be.

—KRISTEN SWANSON, R.N., PH.D., F.A.A.N.

Appendix A

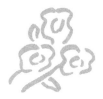

Glossary

DEFINED HERE ARE TERMS USED IN THIS BOOK THAT MAY BE UNFAMILIAR TO some readers. Words that are in **boldface** in a definition are also defined in the glossary.

ANENCEPHALY—A **neural tube defect** in which the brain does not develop and a baby is born with only a brain stem. This condition is incompatible with life.

ANEUPLOIDY—The condition of having more or less than the normal number of chromosomes inside a cell's nucleus, usually because of errors in cell division. A frequent cause of miscarriage.

ANTIPHOSPHOLIPID SYNDROME—A condition in which a person has antibodies to certain fatty acids in the blood, and which is associated with an increased risk of miscarriage. It is also known as Hughes syndrome.

BICORNUATE UTERUS—A uterus formed with two separate compartments, because of a problem in the woman's prenatal development. This malformation can increase the risk of miscarriage or **incompetent cervix.**

BIOCHEMICAL PREGNANCY—In a biochemical pregnancy, a sperm and egg meet, and conception occurs, but the egg does not implant properly in the uterus. Blood and urine tests for hCG are the only evidence of the pregnancy; the egg never develops to the point that it can be seen on an ultrasound.

BLASTOCYST—The ball of cells that rapidly develops after an egg is fertilized, before it implants and becomes an **embryo.**

CERCLAGE—An operation in which a stitch is placed in the cervix in an attempt to prevent premature dilation.

CHROMOSOMAL ANOMALY—In a developing baby, the wrong number of chromosomes or some type of **translocation** in the chromosomes. Many chromosomal anomalies result in miscarriage because they are not compatible with life.

CHROMOSOMES—The matter inside a cell's nucleus that contains human DNA. Each human being should have 23 pairs of chromosomes, for a total of 46. Many genetic diseases result from abnormal numbers of chromosomes, defects in chromosomes, or other errors in cell division.

CORTISOL—A hormone whose production in the body increases in stressful conditions.

D&C (DILATION AND CURETTAGE)—An operation that involves surgically emptying the uterus. This operation is often done to speed the miscarriage process after a miscarriage has been diagnosed.

DIDELPHIC UTERUS—A double uterus, formed because of an error in prenatal development. This malformation can increase the risk of miscarriage.

ECTOPIC PREGNANCY—The condition in which a fertilized egg implants and develops someplace within the body outside of the uterus, usually within one of the fallopian tubes. An ectopic pregnancy can never result in a live birth, and it can be life-threatening to the mother.

EMBRYO—The developing baby from implantation to the end of the eighth week of pregnancy.

ENDOMETRIOSIS—A condition in which endometrial tissue occurs in places in the body outside of the uterus.

ENDOMETRIUM—The lining of the uterus.

FETUS—The developing baby from the end of the eighth week of pregnancy until birth.

FIBROIDS—Growths of tissue on the uterine wall that may be associated with increased miscarriage rates and that can cause pain with menstruation.

FSH (follicle-stimulating hormone)—The hormone that signals the ovaries to begin maturing an egg.

GESTATIONAL SAC—The sac in which a baby develops that is implanted in the uterus.

GESTATIONAL TROPHOBLASTIC DISEASE—A condition in which an egg that carries no chromosomes is fertilized or a normal egg is fertilized by two sperm. After implantation, the egg develops not into a baby but into a "mole," which can become cancerous. This is also called a molar pregnancy.

HABITUAL ABORTION—A once-common medical term for **recurrent miscarriage.**

HCG—See **human chorionic gonadotropin.**

HOLISTIC MEDICINE—An approach to medical care that treats the entire person and focuses on root causes for illnesses rather than just the symptoms.

HOMEOPATHY—A controversial medical practice that involves administering minute amounts of substances that in large doses cause disease symptoms, in order to cure diseases with similar symptoms.

HOMOCYSTEINE—An amino acid whose elevation in the blood may be associated with blood clots and cardiovascular risks.

HUMAN CHORIONIC GONADOTROPIN (hCG)—A hormone that, in the early stages of pregnancy, usually doubles in serum levels every two to three days, although in some viable pregnancies it increases as little as 66 percent over a two-day period. The hCG serum level continues to rise throughout the first trimester. This hormone is the substance that home pregnancy tests detect in confirming pregnancy.

HYDATIDIFORM MOLE—The tissue mass that develops when two sperm fertilize a single egg or one sperm fertilizes an egg with no chromosomes. This tissue mass cannot develop into a baby, and surgery is necessary to remove it. See also **gestational trophoblastic disease.**

HYPERPROLACTINEMIA—A condition in which the hormone **prolactin** is elevated above normal levels in the body and a milky discharge may come from the nipples, even though the woman isn't breastfeeding and hasn't breastfed recently. This condition can be associated with miscarriage.

HYSTEROSALPINGOGRAM—A diagnostic test that involves injecting dye into the uterus and fallopian tubes and then using X-ray imaging to check for abnormalities and blockages of the tubes.

HYSTEROSCOPY—A diagnostic test that involves inserting a scope through a woman's cervix, while she is under anesthesia, and examining her uterus for abnormalities.

INCOMPETENT CERVIX—A cervix that begins to dilate before a baby is ready to be born. This can result in second-trimester miscarriage or preterm birth.

INCOMPLETE MISCARRIAGE/ABORTION—When a woman does not pass all the tissue from a miscarried pregnancy, which can cause continued bleeding and pose a risk of infection. A **D&C** is often recommended in this situation.

KARYOTYPE—An individual's complete set of chromosomes, which can be determined by examining sample cells. To locate any **chromosomal abnormalities,** the cells may be taken from a fetus in the womb (through chorionic villus sampling or amniocentesis), a miscarried baby, or the baby's parents.

LAPAROSCOPY—A diagnostic test in which a small incision is made in a woman's abdomen and a scope is inserted to check for problems.

LH (LUTEINIZING HORMONE)—The hormone that spikes around the time of ovulation.

LUTEAL-PHASE DEFECT—A condition in which the hormones of the second half of the menstrual cycle are inadequate to maintain proper uterine conditions to support a pregnancy. Also called luteal-phase deficiency.

META-ANALYSIS—A scientific study that involves combining several smaller studies to create a sample size large enough to draw conclusions more accurate than those of the smaller studies.

MISOPROSTOL—A medication sometimes used to speed up an **incomplete miscarriage** or **missed miscarriage** for women who wish to avoid a **D&C** but do not want to wait out a natural miscarriage.

MISSED MISCARRIAGE/ABORTION—A medical term for when a baby stops growing in the uterus and no heartbeat can be detected, but vaginal bleeding has yet to start.

MOLAR PREGNANCY—See **gestational trophoblastic disease.**

MYOMECTOMY—Surgical removal of **fibroids.**

NEURAL TUBE DEFECTS—Problems in the development of the spinal cord and brain.

POLYCYSTIC OVARIAN SYNDROME—A condition characterized by multiple cysts on the ovaries and hormonal imbalances, and which is associated with an elevated risk of miscarriage.

Preimplantation genetic diagnosis—A procedure used with in vitro fertilization, in which one cell is removed from the embryo and analyzed for common chromosomal problems that might lead to miscarriage or genetic diseases.

Progesterone—A hormone of the female menstrual cycle that is elevated in the second half of the cycle and helps to sustain the uterine lining for pregnancy. Low progesterone levels may be related to miscarriage.

Prolactin—A hormone that in pregnancy signals the development of the breasts for lactation and after birth signals the breasts to begin producing milk. Elevated prolactin levels before pregnancy are associated with difficulty conceiving, miscarriage, and other medical problems.

Recurrent miscarriage—The condition of having had multiple miscarriages. Some practitioners use this term after two miscarriages, others only after three.

Septate uterus—A uterine abnormality, resulting from a problem in the woman's prenatal development, in which a fibrous membrane, or septum, divides the uterus into two cavities. This condition, which can increase the risk of miscarriage, can be corrected surgically.

Spina bifida—A **neural tube defect** in which the baby's spine does not close properly during the first month of pregnancy. This condition often results in neurological disorders that can range from mild to severe.

Spontaneous abortion—A medical term for miscarriage.

Suppository—A type of medication that is inserted into the vagina or rectum.

Threatened miscarriage/abortion—Any instance of vaginal bleeding in pregnancy. In many cases the pregnancy continues normally.

Thrombophilia—A condition characterized by an abnormal tendency to form blood clots.

Translocation—A condition in which sections of chromosomes have broken off and attached to other chromosomes. This asymptomatic condition, in either parent, can increase a couple's risk of miscarriage, because dividing cells could be missing pieces of chromosomes.

Triploidy—The condition of having three copies of one chromosome instead of two.

Unicornuate uterus—A condition in which one of a woman's fallopian tubes has developed abnormally, resulting in a horn-like deformity on one side of the uterus. If a fertilized egg implants inside the horn, the pregnancy carries the same risks as an **ectopic pregnancy.** The condition is often associated with an **incompetent cervix.**

Uterine lining—The rich mass of tissue and blood vessels that provides nourishment to a developing baby. Also known as the **endometrium.**

Venipuncture—The act of drawing blood from a vein for a laboratory test.

Viable fetus—Describes a developing baby who, if born immediately, would have a chance of survival outside of the womb.

Zygote—A fertilized ovum, before the single cell starts dividing.

Appendix B

Helpful Online Resources

MUCH AS I'D LIKE IT TO BE, this book can't be all things to all people. I've included this appendix in case you want additional information about some topics, such as how to find a support group or a doctor. Be aware that Web addresses can change at any time.

GENERAL INFORMATION ON MISCARRIAGE

After Miscarriage companion Web site (www.aftermiscarriage.com)
BellaOnline (www.miscarriage.bellaonline.com)
Facts About Miscarriage: Information, Healing, and Hope
    (www.pregnancyloss.info)
Empty Cradles (www.empty-cradles.com)
Miscarriage Help (www.miscarriagehelp.com)
Our Miscarriage (www.ourmiscarriage.com)
Silent Grief (www.silentgrief.com)
Miscarriage Association of the United Kingdom
    (www.miscarriageassociation.org.uk)

FORUMS ON PREGNANCY LOSS

Born Angels (www.bornangels.com)
Babyloss (www.babyloss.com)
Multiple Miscarriages Online Support Center
    (www.surrogacy.com/online_support/mm/)

SUPPORT ORGANIZATIONS FOR PREGNANCY LOSS

Share Pregnancy & Infant Loss Support (www.nationalshareoffice.com)
RESOLVE: The National Infertility Association (www.resolve.org)
Miscarriage Association of the United Kingdom
    (www.miscarriageassociation.org.uk)
Save the Baby (www.save-the-baby.com)
Mommies Enduring Neonatal Death (www.mend.org)
HopeXchange (www.hopexchange.com)

A Butterfly's Touch (www.abutterflystouch.org)
Hygeia Foundation (www.hygeia.org)

JEWELRY, GIFTS, AND OTHER MISCARRIAGE MEMORIAL PRODUCTS

Baby Loss Comfort (www.babylosskit.com)
Pregnancy Loss Ribbons (www.pregnancylossribbons.com)
My Forever Child (www.myforeverchild.com)
Little Angels Online (www.littleangelsonlinestore.com)
La Belle Dame (www.labelledame.com)
Earth Mama Angel Baby (www.earthmamaangelbaby.com)

CONDITIONS RELATED TO MISCARRIAGE

Genetic Translocations

MedlinePlus: Translocation
(www.nlm.nih.gov/medlineplus/ency/article/002330.htm)

Polycystic Ovarian Syndrome

SoulCysters (www.soulcysters.com)
Polycystic Ovarian Syndrome Association (www.pcosupport.org)

Infertility

InterNational Council on Infertility Information Dissemination (www.inciid.org)
About Infertility (infertility.about.com)
American Fertility Association (www.theafa.org)

Thyroid Problems

American Thyroid Association (www.thyroid.org)
About Thyroid Disease (thyroid.about.com)
Thyroid Foundation of America (www.tsh.org)
Thyroid Disease Manager (www.thyroidmanager.org)

Ectopic Pregnancy

Ectopic Pregnancy Trust (www.ectopic.org.uk)
Ectopic Pregnancy (www.ectopicpregnancy.com)

Endometriosis

Endometriosis.org (www.endometriosis.org)
EndometriosisZone (www.endozone.org)
Endometriosis Research Center (www.endocenter.org)
Endo-Online: The Voice of the Endometriosis Association
(www.endometriosisassn.org)

Uterine Anomalies

Unicornuate uterus (home.earthlink.net/~hrair/introuni.html)
Congenital Uterine Anomalies Home Page
   (www.wegrokit.com/uterineanomalies/index.htm)
MullerianAnomalies Yahoo Group
   (health.groups.yahoo.com/group/MullerianAnomalies/)
Asherman's Syndrome Online Community (www.ashermans.org)

Misdiagnosed Miscarriage

Misdiagnosed Miscarriage (www.misdiagnosedmiscarriage.com)

Hereditary Thrombophilia

Factor V Leiden Thrombophilia Support Page (www.fvleiden.org)
Protein S Deficiency and Thrombophilia (www.protein.org.uk)

MTHFR and Homocysteine

MTHFR (mthfr.net)
Homocysteine (www.medicinenet.com/homocysteine/article.htm)

Antiphospholipid Syndrome

Hughes Syndrome Foundation (www.hughes-syndrome.org)
Antiphospholipid Antibody Syndrome Resource (apls.tk)

Reproductive Immunology

Reproductive Immunology Support Group (health.groups.yahoo.com/group/
   immunologysupport/)
Is Your Body Baby-friendly? (www.babyfriendlybook.com)
American Society for Reproductive Immunology (www.theasri.org)
A Complete Guide to Reproductive Immunology
   (www.sharedjourney.com/imm.html)

Celiac Disease

Celiac Disease Foundation (www.celiac.org)
Celiac Disease and Gluten-free Diet Support Center (www.celiac.com)
Celiac Sprue Association (www.csaceliacs.org)
University of Maryland Center for Celiac Research (celiaccenter.org)

Conditions Incompatible with Life

A Heartbreaking Choice (www.aheartbreakingchoice.com)
Anencephaly Net (www.anencephaly.net)
Trisomy 18 Foundation (www.trisomy18support.org)
Support Organization for Trisomy 18, 13, and Related Disorders
   (www.trisomy.org)

Blighted Ovum

Coping with Pregnancy Loss (blightedovum.kokopuff.net)

ADOPTION

About.com: Adoption/Foster Care (adoption.about.com)
Adoption.com (www.adoption.com)
National Adoption Center (www.adopt.org)
The Adoption Guide (www.theadoptionguide.com)

SURROGACY

American Surrogacy Center (www.surrogacy.com)
All About Surrogacy (www.allaboutsurrogacy.com)
Everything Surrogacy (www.everythingsurrogacy.com)

TRYING TO CONCEIVE

Temperature Charting

MyMonthlyCycles (www.mymonthlycycles.com)
Ovusoft (www.ovusoft.com)
FertilityFriend (www.fertilityfriend.com)
WebWomb (www.webwomb.com)

Trying-to-Conceive (TTC) Support Groups

TTC–After Multiple Miscarriages (talk.sheknows.com/forumdisplay.php?f=58)
TTC After Recurrent Miscarriage (gynosaur.com/phorum/list.php?f=5)
TTC After Miscarriage (messageboards.ivillage.com/iv-ppttcmiss)
Trying to Conceive International (www.tryingtoconceive.com)

Inexpensive Pregnancy and Ovulation Tests

Save On Tests (www.saveontests.com)
AccuratePregnancyTests.com (www.accuratepregnancytests.com)
BabyHopes (www.babyhopes.com)
Craig Medical (www.craigmedical.com/pregnancy_tests.htm)
Pregnancy Test Store (www.pregnancyteststore.com)

Doctor Search

American Society for Reproductive Medicine (www.asrm.org)
Society for Reproductive Endocrinology and Infertility (www.socrei.org)

PREGNANCY AFTER MISCARRIAGE

Pregnancy-After-Miscarriage Support Groups

Subsequent Pregnancy After a Loss Support (www.spals.com)

Doppler Rental

Stork Radio (www.storkradio.com)
BabyBeat (www.babybeat.com)
HearTones (www.heartones.com)
Dynamic Doppler (www.dynamicdoppler.com)

DIET, SUPPLEMENTS, AND HERBAL MEDICINE

Healthy Diet

MyPyramid Eating Plan (www.mypyramid.gov)
U.S. Department of Health & Human Services A Healthy Diet Plan
(www.4woman.gov/faq/diet.htm)

Nutritional Supplements

What's in the Bottle? An Introduction to Dietary Supplements
(www.nccam.nih.gov/health/bottle)
U.S. Food and Drug Administration: Dietary Supplements Overview
(www.cfsan.fda.gov/~dms/supplmnt.html)
NutritionalSupplements.com (www.nutritionalsupplements.com)

Herbs

Herbal Medicine Materia Medica (www.healthy.net; select "Herbal Medicine" and
then "Materia Medica")

Weight Loss

Weight Watchers (www.weightwatchers.com)

LESBIANS AND MISCARRIAGE

University of California, San Francisco, Lesbian Health & Research Center
(www.lesbianhealthinfo.org)

SUPPORT FOR SINGLE MOTHERS

SingleRose (www.singlerose.com)
Single Parents Network online forum
(www.singlefamilyvoices.com/eve/forums)
National Organization of Single Mothers (www.singlemothers.org)

References

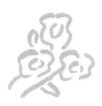

CHAPTER 1

Some Basic Facts About Miscarriage

Brigham, S. A., C. Conlon, and R. G. Farquharson. "A longitudinal study of pregnancy outcome following idiopathic recurrent miscarriage." *Human Reproduction* 14 (November 1999): 2868–71.

U.S. National Library of Medicine and National Institutes of Health. "Abortion—threatened." *MedlinePlus.* http://www.nlm.nih.gov/medlineplus/ency/article/000907.htm.

A Quick Guide to Miscarriage Terms

Brigham, S. A., C. Conlon, and R. G. Farquharson. "A longitudinal study of pregnancy outcome following idiopathic recurrent miscarriage." *Human Reproduction* 14 (November 1999): 2868–71.

Creighton University Medical Center. "Basic imaging: ultrasound of early pregnancy." http://radiology.creighton.edu/pregnancy.htm#section4.

The D&C Question

Ballagh, S. A., H. A. Harris, and K. Demasio. "Is curettage needed for uncomplicated incomplete spontaneous abortion?" *American Journal of Obstetrics and Gynecology* 179 (November 1998): 1279–82.

Nonsurgical Miscarriages

Trinder, J., et al. "Management of miscarriage: expectant, medical, or surgical? Results of randomised controlled trial (miscarriage treatment [MIST] trial)." *British Medical Journal* 332 (May 2006): 1235–40.

Ectopic Pregnancies

Ramakrishnan, K., and D. C. Schneid. "Ectopic pregnancy: expectant management or immediate surgery? An algorithm to improve outcomes." *Journal of Family Practice* 56 (June 2006): 517–22.

U.S. National Library of Medicine and National Institutes of Health. "Ectopic pregnancy." *MedlinePlus.* http://www.nlm.nih.gov/medlineplus/ency/article/000895.htm.

CHAPTER 2

Unlikely Causes of Miscarriage

Henriksen, T. B., et al. "Alcohol consumption at the time of conception and spontaneous abortion." *American Journal of Epidemiology* 160 (2004): 661–67.

Hjollund, N. H., et al. "Spontaneous abortion and physical strain around implantation: a follow-up study of first-pregnancy planners." *Epidemiology* 11 (January 2000): 18–23.

Khanna, N. "Effects of exercise on pregnancy." *American Family Physician* 57 (April 1998): 1770–2.

Klonoff-Cohen, H., P. Lam-Kruglick, and C. Gonzalez. "Effects of maternal and paternal alcohol consumption on the success rates of in vitro fertilization and gamete intrafallopian transfer." *Fertility and Sterility* 79 (February 2003): 330–39.

Lass, A., et al. "The effect of endometrial polyps on outcomes of in vitro fertilization (IVF) cycles." *Journal of Assisted Reproduction and Genetics* 16 (September 1999): 410–15.

Li, D., L. Liu, and R. Odouli. "Exposure to nonsteroidal anti-inflammatory drugs during pregnancy and risk of miscarriage: population-based cohort study." *British Medical Journal* 327 (2003): 368.

McDonald, A. D., et al. "Spontaneous abortion and occupation." *Journal of Occupational Medicine* 28 (December 1986): 1232–8.

Nielsen, G. L., et al. "Risk of adverse birth outcome and miscarriage in pregnant users of nonsteroidal anti-inflammatory drugs: population-based observational study and case-control study." *British Medical Journal* 322 (February 2001): 266–70.

Pérez-Medina, T., et al. "Endometrial polyps and their implication in the pregnancy rates of patients undergoing intrauterine insemination: a prospective, randomized study." *Human Reproduction* 20 (2005): 1632–35.

U.S. National Library of Medicine and National Institutes of Health. "Asherman's syndrome." *MedlinePlus*. http://www.nlm.nih.gov/medlineplus/ency/article/001483.htm.

Walpole, I., S. Zubrick, and J. Pontre. "Confounding variables in studying the effects of maternal alcohol consumption before and during pregnancy." *Journal of Epidemiology and Community Health* 43 (1989): 153–61.

Windham, G. C., et al. "Moderate maternal alcohol consumption and risk of spontaneous abortion." *Epidemiology* 8 (1997): 509.

Chromosomal Anomalies

Bove, F., Y. Shim, and P. Zeitz. "Drinking water contaminants and adverse pregnancy outcomes: a review." *Environmental Health Perspectives* 110 (February 2002): 61–74.

Bricker, L., and R. G. Farquharson. "Types of pregnancy loss in recurrent miscarriage: implications for research and clinical practice." *Human Reproduction* 17 (May 2002): 1345–50.

Campana, M., A. Serra, and G. Neri. "Role of chromosome aberrations in recurrent abortion: a study of 269 balanced translocations." *American Journal of Medical Genetics* 24 (June 1986): 341–56.

De la Chica, R., et al. "Chromosomal instability in amniocytes from fetuses of mothers who smoke." *Journal of the American Medical Association* 293 (2005): 1212–22.

De La Rochebrochard, E., and P. Thonneau. "Paternal age and maternal age are risk factors for miscarriage: results of a multicentre European study." *Human Reproduction* 17 (June 2002): 1649–56.

Franssen, M. T. M., et al. "Reproductive outcome after chromosome analysis in couples with two or more miscarriages: index-control study." *British Medical Journal* 332 (April 2006): 759–63.

Hassold, T., and D. Chui. "Maternal age-specific rates of numerical chromosome abnormalities with special reference to trisomy." *Human Genetics* 70 (1985): 11–17.

Henriksen, T. B., et al. "Alcohol consumption at the time of conception and spontaneous abortion." *American Journal of Epidemiology* 160 (2004): 661–67.

Li, D., et al. "A population-based prospective cohort study of personal exposure to magnetic fields during pregnancy and the risk of miscarriage." *Epidemiology* 13 (January 2002): 9–20.

Ljunger, E., et al. "Chromosomal anomalies in first-trimester miscarriages." *Acta Obstetricia et Gynecologica Scandinavica* 84 (November 1995): 1103.

MacNair, T. "Translocation." *Bbc.co.uk Health.* http://www.bbc.co.uk/health/conditions/chromosomaltranslocation1.shtml.

Mailhes, J. B., et al. "Electromagnetic fields enhance chemically induced hyperploidy in mammalian oocytes." *Mutagenesis* (1997): 347–51.

Nasseri, A., et al. "Elevated day 3 serum follicle-stimulating hormone and/or estradiol may predict fetal aneuploidy." *Fertility and Sterility* 71 (April 1999): 715–18.

Robbins, W. A., et al. "Effect of lifestyle exposures on sperm aneuploidy." *Cytogenetic and Genome Research* 111 (2005): 371–77.

Rubes, J., et al. "Episodic air pollution is associated with increased DNA fragmentation in human sperm without other changes in semen quality." *Human Reproduction* 20 (June 2005): 2776–83.

Rubio, C., et al. "Chromosomal abnormalities and embryo development in recurrent miscarriage couples." *Human Reproduction* 18 (January 2003): 182–88.

Salim, R., et al. "A comparative study of the morphology of congenital uterine anomalies in women with and without a history of recurrent first-trimester miscarriage." *Human Reproduction* 18 (January 2003): 162–66.

Shaw, G. M., and L. A. Croen. "Human adverse reproductive outcomes and electromagnetic field exposures: review of epidemiologic studies." *Environmental Health Perspectives* 101 (December 1993): 107–19.

Slama, R., et al. "Influence of paternal age on the risk of spontaneous abortion." *American Journal of Epidemiology* 161 (2005): 816–23.

Sullivan, A. E., et al. "Recurrent fetal aneuploidy and recurrent miscarriage." *Obstetrics & Gynecology* 104 (2004): 784–88.

Šutiaková, Irena, et al. "Chromosome damage in peripheral lymphocytes of sheep induced by chlorine in drinking water." *International Journal of Environmental Health Research* 14 (October 2005): 381–90.

University of Utah Genetic Science Learning Center. "Robertsonian translocation." *Learn.Genetics.* http://learn.genetics.utah.edu/units/disorders/karyotype/robertsonian.cfm.

Vorsanova, S. G., et al. "Evidence for high frequency of chromosomal mosaicism in spontaneous abortions revealed by iInterphase FISH analysis." *Journal of Histochemistry and Cytochemistry* 53 (2005): 375–80.

Xu, X., et al. "Association of petrochemical exposure with spontaneous abortion." *Occupational and Environmental Medicine* 55 (1998): 31–36.

Infections

Donders, G. G., et al. "Relationship of bacterial vaginosis and mycoplasmas to the risk of spontaneous abortion." *American Journal of Obstetrics and Gynecology* 183 (August 2000): 431–37.

Ralph, S. G., et al. "Influence of bacterial vaginosis on conception and miscarriage in the first trimester: cohort study." *British Medical Journal* 319 (July 1999): 220–23.

U.S. Centers for Disease Control and Prevention. "Bacterial vaginosis—CDC Fact Sheet." http://www.cdc.gov/std/bv/STDFact-Bacterial-Vaginosis.htm.

Waites, K. B. "Ureaplasma infection." *eMedicine.* http://www.emedicine.com/med/topic2340.htm.

Anatomical Problems with the Uterus

Bajekal, N., and T. C. Li. "Fibroids, infertility, and pregnancy wastage." *Human Reproduction Update* 6 (2000): 614–20.

Cleveland Clinic. "Facts about endometriosis." *The Cleveland Clinic Health Information Center.* http://www.clevelandclinic.org/health/health-info/docs/1100/1119.asp?index=5751.

Gaucherand, P., et al. "Obstetrical prognosis of the septate uterus: a plea for treatment of the septum." *European Journal of Obstetrics, Gynecology, and Reproductive Biology* 54 (April 1994): 109–12.

Grimbizis, G., et al. "Hysteroscopic septum resection in patients with recurrent abortions or infertility." *Human Reproduction* 13 (1998): 1188–93.

Herbst, A. L., et al. "A comparison of pregnancy experience in DES-exposed and DES-unexposed daughters." *Journal of Reproductive Medicine* 24 (February 1980): 62–69.

Hunter, R. H. F. "Tubal ectopic pregnancy: a patho-physiological explanation involving endometriosis." *Human Reproduction* 17 (July 2002): 1688–91.

Kupesic, S., A. Kurjak, S. Skenderovic, and D. Bjelos. "Screening for uterine abnormalities by three-dimensional ultrasound improves perinatal outcome." *Journal of Perinatal Medicine* 30 (2002): 9–17.

Li, T. C., R. Mortimer, and I. D. Cooke. "Myomectomy: a retrospective study to examine reproductive performance before and after surgery." *Human Reproduction* 14 (July 1999): 1735–40.

Lin, P. C. "Reproductive outcomes in women with uterine anomalies." *Journal of Women's Health* 13 (January 2004): 33–39.

Matorras, R., et al. "Endometriosis and spontaneous abortion rate: a cohort study in infertile women." *European Journal of Obstetrics, Gynecology, and Reproductive Biology* 77 (March 1998): 101–5.

National Uterine Fibroids Foundation. "Statistics." http://www.nuff.org/health_statistics.htm.

National Women's Health Information Center. "Endometriosis." *Womenshealth.gov.* http://www.4woman.gov/faq/endomet.htm.

National Women's Health Information Center. "Uterine fibroids." *Womenshealth.gov.* http://www.4woman.gov/faq/fibroids.htm.

Pritts, E. A. "Fibroids and infertility: a systematic review of the evidence." *Obstetrical & Gynecological Survey* 56 (August 2001): 483–91.

Raga, F., et al. "Reproductive impact of congenital Mullerian anomalies." *Human Reproduction* 12 (1997): 2277–81.

Rooney, B., and B. C. Calhoun. "Induced abortion and risk of later premature births." *Journal of American Physicians and Surgeons* 8 (Summer 2003): 46–49.

Shands HealthCare. "Special-care pregnancies." *Pregnancy Health Center.* http://www.shands.org/health/pregnancy/specialcare/articles/cervix.html.

Valli, E., et al. "Hysteroscopic metroplasty improves gestational outcome in women with recurrent spontaneous abortion." *Journal of the American Association of Gynecologic Laparoscopists* 11 (May 2004): 240–44.

Weiss, A., E. Shalev, and S. Romano. "Hysteroscopy may be justified after two miscarriages." *Human Reproduction* 20 (May 2005): 2628–31.

Wheeler, J. M., B. M. Johnston, and L. R. Malinak. "The relationship of endometriosis to spontaneous abortion." *Fertility & Sterility* 39 (May 1983): 656–60.

Hormonal Imbalances

Abalovich, M., et al. "Overt and subclinical hypothyroidism complicating pregnancy." *Thyroid* 12 (January 2002): 63–68.

American Society for Reproductive Medicine. "Patient's fact sheet: prolactin excess." http://www.asrm.org/Patients/FactSheets/Prolactin_Excess-Fact.pdf.

Balen, A. H., et al. "Miscarriage rates following in vitro fertilization are increased in women with polycystic ovaries and reduced by pituitary desensitization with buserelin." *Human Reproduction* 8 (1993): 959–64.

Balen, A. H., S. Tan, and H. S. Jacobs. "Hypersecretion of luteinising hormone: a significant cause of infertility and miscarriage." *British Journal of Obstetrics & Gynecology* 100 (December 1993): 1082.

Craig, L. B., R. W. Ke, and W. H. Kutteh. "Increased prevalence of insulin resistance in women with a history of recurrent pregnancy loss." *Fertility & Sterility* 78 (September 2002): 487–90.

Doldi, N., et al. "Polycystic ovary syndrome: anomalies in progesterone production." *Human Reproduction* 13 (1998): 290–93.

Dendrinos, S., et al. "Thyroid autoimmunity in patients with recurrent spontaneous miscarriages." *Gynecology & Endocrinology* 14 (August 2000): 270–74.

Esplin, M., et al. "Thyroid autoantibodies are not associated with recurrent pregnancy loss." *American Journal of Obstetrics and Gynecology* 179 (December 1998): 1583–86.

Fedorcsák, Péter, et al. "The impact of obesity and insulin resistance on the outcome of IVF or ICSI in women with polycystic ovarian syndrome." *Human Reproduction* 16 (June 2001): 1086–91.

Glueck, C. J., et al. "Plasminogen activator inhibitor activity: an independent risk factor for the high miscarriage rate during pregnancy in women with polycystic ovary syndrome." *Metabolism* 48 (December 1999): 1589–95.

Heindel, J. J. "Endocrine disruptors and the obesity epidemic." *Toxicological Sciences* 76 (2003): 247–49.

Hirahara, F., et al. "Hyperprolactinemic recurrent miscarriage and results of randomized bromocriptine treatment trials." *Fertility & Sterility* 70 (August 1998): 253–55.

Homburg, R., et al. "Influence of serum luteinising hormone concentrations on ovulation, conception, and early pregnancy loss in polycystic ovary syndrome." *British Medical Journal* 297 (October 1988): 1024–26.

Jones, G. S. "Luteal-phase defect: a review of pathophysiology." *Current Opinions in Obstetrics & Gynecology* 3 (October 1991): 641–48.

National Women's Health Information Center. "Polycystic Ovarian Syndrome." *Womenshealth.gov.* http://www.4woman.gov/faq/pcos.htm.

Prummel, M. F., et al. "Thyroid autoimmunity and miscarriage." *European Journal of Endocrinology* 150 (2004): 751–55.

Regan, L., E. J. Owen, and H. S. Jacobs. "Hypersecretion of luteinising hormone, infertility, and miscarriage." *Lancet* 336 (November 1990): 1141–44.

Rossi, A. M., S. Vilska, and P. K. Heinonen. "Outcome of pregnancies in women with treated or untreated hyperprolactinemia." *European Journal of Obstetrics, Gynecology, and Reproductive Biology* 63 (December 1995): 143–46.

Rushworth, F. H., et al. "Prospective pregnancy outcome in untreated recurrent miscarriers with thyroid autoantibodies." *Human Reproduction* 15 (July 2000): 1637–39.

Stagnaro-Green, A., and D. Glinoer. "Thyroid autoimmunity and the risk of miscarriage." *Best Practice & Research Clinical Endocrinology & Metabolism* 18 (June 2004): 167–81.

Watson, H., et al.. "Hypersecretion of luteinizing hormone and ovarian steroids in women with recurrent early miscarriage." *Human Reproduction* 8 (June 1993): 829–33.

Youngerman-Cole, S. "Progesterone." *A–Z Health Guide from WebMD: Medical Tests.* http://www.webmd.com/hw/healthy_women/hw42146.asp.

Blood-clotting Disorders

Bare, S. N., et al. "Factor V Leiden as a risk factor for miscarriage and reduced fertility." *Australia and New Zealand Journal of Obstetrics and Gynaecology* 40 (May 2000): 186–90.

Bertolaccini, M. L., et al. "Antiphospholipid antibody tests: spreading the net." *Annals of the Rheumatic Diseases* 64 (April 2005): 1639–43.

Bick, R. L., and D. Hoppensteadt. "Thrombohemorrhagic defects and recurrent miscarriage syndrome." *Blood* 104 (2004): 2602.

Carp, H., et al. "Hereditary thrombophilias are not associated with a decreased live birth rate in women with recurrent miscarriage." *Fertility & Sterility* 78 (July 2002): 58–62.

Carp, H., et al. "Prevalence of genetic markers for thrombophilia in recurrent pregnancy loss." *Human Reproduction* 17 (June 2002): 1633–37.

Carsons, S., and E. Belilos. "Antiphospholipid syndrome." *Emedicine from WebMD.* http://www.emedicine.com/med/topic2923.htm.

Di Nisio, M., L. W. Peters, and S. Middeldorp. "Anticoagulants for the treatment of recurrent pregnancy loss in women without antiphospholipid syndrome." *The Cochrane Library* 2 (2006).

Empson, M., et al. "Prevention of recurrent miscarriage for women with antiphospholipid antibody or lupus anticoagulant." *Cochrane Database of Systemic Reviews* 2 (2006).

Foka, Z. J., et al. "Factor V Leiden and prothrombin G20210A mutations, but not methylenetetrahydrofolate reductase C677T, are associated with recurrent miscarriages." *Human Reproduction* 15 (February 2000): 458–62.

Fujimura, H., et al. "Common C677T polymorphism in the methylenetetrahydrofolate reductase gene increases the risk for deep vein thrombosis in patients with predisposition of thrombophilia." *Thrombosis Research* 98 (April 2000): 1–8.

Holmes, Z. R., et al. "The C677T MTHFR gene mutation is not predictive of risk for recurrent fetal loss." *British Journal of Haematology* 105 (April 1999): 98–101.

Hoppensteadt, D., et al. "Hyperhomocysteinemia in cancer patients with thrombosis is not associated with methylenetetrahydrofolate reductase (MTHFR) gene mutations and can be down regulated by low molecular weight heparin (LMWHs) treatment." *Journal of Clinical Oncology* 23 (June 2005): 2056.

Jacques, P. F., et al. "Relation between folate status, a common mutation in methylenetetrahydrofolate reductase, and plasma homocysteine concentrations." *Circulation* 93 (1996): 7–9.

Jivraj, S., R. Rai, J. Underwood, and L. Regan. "Genetic thrombophilic mutations among couples with recurrent miscarriage." *Human Reproduction Advance Access* (January 2006): 1161–5.

Key, N. S., and R. C. McGlennen. "Hyperhomocyst(e)inemia and thrombophilia." *Archives of Pathology and Laboratory Medicine* 126 (2002): 1367–75.

McIntire, J. A. "Antiphospholipid antibodies in implantation failures." *American Journal of Reproductive Immunology* 49 (April 2003): 221–29.

Nelen, W., et al. "Maternal homocysteine and chorionic vascularization in recurrent early pregnancy loss." *Human Reproduction* 15 (April 2000): 954–60.

Nelen, W. L., et al. "Methylenetetrahydrofolate reductase polymorphism affects the change in homocysteine and folate concentrations resulting from low dose folic acid supplementation in women with unexplained recurrent miscarriages." *Journal of Nutrition* 128 (August 1998): 1336–41.

Pauer, H. U., et al. "Factor XII deficiency is strongly associated with primary recurrent abortions." *Fertility & Sterility* 80 (September 2003): 590–94.

Quenby, S., et al.. "Recurrent miscarriage and long-term thrombosis risk: a case-control study." *Human Reproduction* 20 (March 2005): 1729–32.

Quéré, I., et al. "A woman with five consecutive fetal deaths: case report and retrospective analysis of hyperhomocysteinemia prevalence in 100 consecutive women with recurrent miscarriages." *Fertility & Sterility* 69 (January 1998): 152–54.

Quéré, I., et al. "Vitamin supplementation and pregnancy outcome in women with recurrent early pregnancy loss and hyperhomocysteinemia." *Fertility & Sterility* 75 (April 2001): 823–25.

Rai, R. S. "Antiphospholipid syndrome and recurrent miscarriage." *Journal of Postgraduate Medicine* 48 (2002): 3–4.

Rey, E., S. R. Kahn, M. David, and I. Shrier. "Thrombophilic disorders and fetal loss: a meta-analysis." *Lancet* 361 (March 2003): 901–8.

Reznikoff-Etiévanta, M. F., et al. "Factor V Leiden and G20210A prothrombin mutations are risk factors for very early recurrent miscarriage." *British Journal of Obstetrics & Gynecology* 108 (December 2001): 1251.

Sarig, G., et al. "Thrombophilia is common in women with idiopathic pregnancy loss and is associated with late pregnancy wastage." *Fertility & Sterility* 77 (February 2002): 342–47.

Sugi, T., et al. "Antiphosphatidylethanolamine antibodies in recurrent early pregnancy loss and mid-to-late pregnancy loss." *Journal of Obstetrics and Gynaecology Research* 30 (August 2004): 326.

Ubbink, J. B., et al. "The effect of a subnormal vitamin B_6 status on homocysteine metabolism." *Journal of Clinical Investigation* 98 (July 1996): 177–84.

Unfried, G., et al. "The C677T polymorphism of the methylenetetrahydrofolate reductase gene and idiopathic recurrent miscarriage." *Obstetrics & Gynecology* 99 (2002): 614–19.

Wang, X. P., et al. "C677T and A1298C mutation of the methylenetetrahydrofolate reductase gene in unexplained recurrent spontaneous abortion." *Zhongua Fu Chan Ke Za Zhi* 39 (April 2004): 238–41.

Zetterberg, H., et al. "Gene-gene interaction between fetal MTHFR 677C>T and transcobalamin 776C>G polymorphisms in human spontaneous abortion." *Human Reproduction* 18 (September 2003): 1948–50.

Zetterberg, H. "Methylenetetrahydrofolate reductase and transcobalamin genetic polymorphisms in human spontaneous abortion: biological and clinical implications." *Reproductive Biology and Endocrinology* 2 (February 2004). http://www.rbej.com/content/2/1/7/.

Zittoun, J., et al. "Plasma homocysteine levels related to interactions between folate status and methylenetetrahydrofolate reductase: a study in 52 healthy subjects." *Metabolism* 47 (November 1998): 1413–18.

Immunological Malfunctions

Abbas, A., et al. "Analysis of human leukocyte antigen (HLA)–G polymorphism in normal women and in women with recurrent spontaneous abortions." *European Journal of Immunogenetics* 31 (December 2004): 275.

Aldrich, C. L., et al. "HLA-G genotypes and pregnancy outcome in couples with unexplained recurrent miscarriages." *Molecular Human Reproduction* 7 (December 2001): 1167–72.

Bainbridge, D., et al. "HLA-G remains a mystery." *Trends in Immunology* 22 (October 2001): 548–52.

Christiansen, O. B., et al. "Association between HLA-DR1 and -DR3 antigens and unexplained repeated miscarriage." *Human Reproduction* Update 5 (1999): 249–55.

Christiansen, O. B., et al. "Histocompatibility antigen studies in women with recurrent miscarriages and Mullerian uterine anomalies." *European Journal of Obstetrics, Gynecology, and Reproductive Biology* 78 (May 1998): 73–7.

Christiansen, O. B., et al. "Studies on associations between human leukocyte antigen (HLA) class II alleles and antiphospholipid antibodies in Danish and Czech women with recurrent miscarriages." *Human Reproduction* 13 (1998): 3326–31.

Emmer, P. M., et al. "Altered phenotype of HLA-G expressing trophoblast and decidual natural killer cells in pathological pregnancies." *Human Reproduction* 17 (April 2002): 1072–80.

Garcia-De La Torre, I., et al. "Prevalence of antinuclear antibodies in patients with habitual abortion and in normal and toxemic pregnancies." *Rheumatology International* 4 (June 1984): 87–89.

Kallen, C. B., and A. Arici. "Immune testing in fertility practice: truth or deception?" *Current Opinion in Obstetrics and Gynecology* 15 (June 2003): 225–31.

Kutteh, W. H. "Antiphospholipid antibody–associated recurrent pregnancy loss: treatment with heparin and low-dose aspirin is superior to low-dose aspirin alone." *American Journal of Obstetrics and Gynecology* 174 (1996): 1584–89.

Ober, C., et al. "The miscarriage-associated HLA-G –725G allele influences transcription rates in JEG-3 cells." *Human Reproduction* 21 (February 2006): 1743–48.

Pfeiffer, K. A., et al. "The HLA-G genotype is potentially associated with idiopathic recurrent spontaneous abortion." *Molecular Human Reproduction* 7 (April 2001): 373–78.

Porter, T. F., et al. "Immunotherapy for recurrent miscarriage." *Cochrane Database of Systemic Reviews* 2 (2006).

Reproductive Immunology Associates. "Miscarriages can be prevented." http://www.rialab.com/miscarriages_prevented.php.

Stricker, R. B., A. Steinleitner, and E. E. Winger. "Intravenous immunoglobulin (IVIg) therapy for immunologic abortion." *Clinical and Applied Immunology Reviews* 2 (2002): 187–99.

U.S. National Library of Medicine. "Natural killer cells." *Genetics Home Reference.* http://ghr.nlm.nih.gov/ghr/glossary/naturalkillercells.

Yamada, H., et al. "Preconceptional natural-killer-cell activity and percentage as predictors of biochemical pregnancy and spontaneous abortion with normal chromosome karyotype." *American Journal of Reproductive Immunology* 50 (October 2003): 351–54.

Yassin, M. "Spotlight on the role of natural killer cells in recurrent spontaneous abortion." *Ain Shams Journal of Obstetrics & Gynecology* 2 (March 2005): 238–39.

Maternal Illness

Bennett, M. "Vitamin B_{12} deficiency, infertility and recurrent fetal loss." *Journal of Reproductive Medicine* 46 (March 2001): 209–12.

Brydon., P., et al. "Pregnancy outcome in women with type 2 diabetes mellitus needs to be addressed." *International Journal of Clinical Practice* 54 (September 2000): 418–19.

Chianchiano, N., et al. "Uteroplacental blood flow in pregnant women with hypertension and recurrent spontaneous abortion." *Acta European Fertility* 22 (May 1991): 151–52.

Combs, C. A., and J. L. Kitzmuller. "Spontaneous abortion and congenital malformations in diabetes." *Baillieres Clinical Obstetrics & Gynaecology* 5 (June 1991): 315–31.

Crowe, A. V., et al. "Pregnancy does not adversely affect renal transplant function." *QJM* 92 (1999): 631–35.

Dahele, A. and S. Ghosh. "Vitamin B_{12} deficiency in untreated celiac disease." *American Journal of Gastroenterology* 96 (March 2001): 745–50.

ESHRE Capri Workshop Group. "Nutrition and reproduction in women." *Human Reproduction Update* 12 (January 2006): 193–207.

Fasano, A., et al. "Prevalence of celiac disease in at-risk and not-at-risk groups in the United States: a large multicenter study." *Archives of Internal Medicine* 163 (February 2003): 286–92.

Gallagher, K. "Methyldopa for chronic hypertension during pregnancy." *Yahoo! Health.* http://health.yahoo.com/ency/healthwise/hw61257.

Gasbarrini, A., et al. "Recurrent spontaneous abortion and intrauterine fetal growth retardation as symptoms of celiac disease." *Lancet* 356 (July 2000): 399–400.

Hallert, C., et al. "Evidence of poor vitamin status in celiac patients on a gluten-free diet for 10 years." *Alimentary Pharmacology & Therapeutics* 16 (July 2002): 1333.

Hawkins, M. M., and R. A. Smith. "Pregnancy outcomes in childhood cancer survivors: probable effects of abdominal irradiation." *International Journal of Cancer* 15 (March 1989): 399–402.

Hou, S. "Pregnancy in women requiring dialysis for renal failure." *American Journal of Kidney Diseases* 9 (April 1987): 368–73.

Lashen, H., K. Fear, and D. W. Sturdee. "Obesity is associated with increased risk of first-trimester and recurrent miscarriage: matched case–control study." *Human Reproduction* 19 (May 2004): 1644–46.

Lockshin, M. D. "Pregnancy and lupus." *Lupus Foundation of America.* http://www.lupus.org/education/brochures/pregnancy.html#4.

Mills, J. L., et al. "Incidence of spontaneous abortion among normal women and insulin-dependent diabetic women whose pregnancies were identified within 21 days of conception." *The New England Journal of Medicine* 319 (December 1988): 1617–23.

Rosenn, B., et al. "Glycemic thresholds for spontaneous abortion and congenital malformations in insulin-dependent diabetes mellitus." *Obstetrics & Gynecology* 84 (1994): 515–20.

Schlumberger, M., et al. "Exposure to radioactive iodine-131 for scintigraphy or therapy does not preclude pregnancy in thyroid cancer patients." *Journal of Nuclear Medicine* 37 (1996): 606–12.

Silverstone, A., et al. "Maternal hypertension and intrauterine fetal death in mid-pregnancy." *British Journal of Obstetrics & Gynecology* 87 (June 1980): 457.

Sorosky, J. I., A. K. Sood, and T. E. Buekers. "The use of chemotherapeutic agents during pregnancy." *Obstetrics and Gynecology Clinics of North America* 24 (September 1997): 591–99.

Tata, L. J., et al. "Fertility and pregnancy-related events in women with celiac disease: a population-based cohort study." *Gastroenterology* 128 (April 2005): 849–55.

Zemlickis, D., et al. "Fetal outcome after in utero exposure to cancer chemotherapy." *Archives of Internal Medicine* 152 (March 1992): 573–76.

Lifestyle Factors

Arck, P. "Stress and embryo implantation." *Journal de Gynécologie Obstétrique et Biologie de la Reproduction* 33 (January 2004): 40–42.

Arck, P. C., et al. "Stress and immune mediators in miscarriage." *Human Reproduction* 16 (July 2001): 1505–11.

Clark, D. A., D. Banwatt, and G. Chaouat. "Stress-triggered abortion in mice prevented by alloimmunization." *American Journal of Reproductive Immunology* 29 (April 1993): 141–47.

Craig, M. "Stress and recurrent miscarriages." *Stress* 4 (2001): 205–13.

Fenster, L., et al. "Psychologic stress in the workplace and spontaneous abortion." *American Journal of Epidemiology* 142 (1995): 1176–83.

Ferraro, F., R. Ferraro, and A. Massard. "Consequences of cocaine addiction during pregnancy on the development in the child." *Archives de Pédiatrie* 4 (July 1997): 677–82.

Giannelli, M., et al. "The effect of caffeine consumption and nausea on the risk of miscarriage." *Paediatric & Perinatal Epidemiology* 17 (October 2003): 316.

Gomes-da-Silva, J., et al. "Prenatal exposure to methamphetamine in the rat." *Annals of the New York Academy of Sciences* 965 (June 2002): 68.

Kline, J., et al. "Smoking: a risk factor for spontaneous abortion." *New England Journal of Medicine* 297 (October 1977): 793–96.

Lindbohm, M. L., M. Sallmen, and H. Taskinen. "Effects of exposure to environmental tobacco smoke on reproductive health." *Scandinavian Journal of Work and Environmental Health* 28 (2002): 84–96.

Milad, M. P., et al. "Stress and anxiety do not result in pregnancy wastage." *Human Reproduction* 13 (1998): 2296–3000.

Nelson, D. B., et al. "Does stress influence early pregnancy loss?" *Annals of Epidemiology* 13 (April 2003): 223–29.

Nepomnaschy, P. A., et al. "Cortisol levels and very early pregnancy loss in humans." *Proceedings of the National Academy of Sciences* 103 (March 2006): 3938–42.

Parazzini, F., et al. "Coffee consumption and risk of hospitalized miscarriage before 12 weeks of gestation." *Human Reproduction* 13 (August 1998): 2286–91.

Sata, F., et al. "Caffeine intake, CYP1A2 polymorphism, and the risk of recurrent pregnancy loss." *Molecular Human Reproduction* 11 (April 2005): 357–60.

Venners, S. A., et al. "Paternal smoking and pregnancy loss: a prospective study using a biomarker of pregnancy." *American Journal of Epidemiology* 159 (2004): 993–1001.

Windham, G. C., et al. "Exposure to environmental and mainstream tobacco smoke and risk of spontaneous abortion." *American Journal of Epidemiology* 149 (1999): 243–47.

Unknown Causes of Miscarriage

Brigham, S. A., C. Conlon, and R. G. Farquharson. "A longitudinal study of pregnancy outcome following idiopathic recurrent miscarriage." *Human Reproduction* 14 (November 1999): 2868–71.

CHAPTER 3

If You've Had More Than One Miscarriage

Brigham, S. A., C. Conlon, and R. G. Farquharson. "A longitudinal study of pregnancy outcome following idiopathic recurrent miscarriage." *Human Reproduction* 14 (November 1999): 2868–71.

Stephenson, M. D. "Frequency of factors associated with habitual abortion in 197 couples." *Fertility and Sterility* 66 (July 1996): 24–29.

A Note on Scientific Proof

Brigham, S. A., C. Conlon, and R. G. Farquharson. "A longitudinal study of pregnancy outcome following idiopathic recurrent miscarriage." *Human Reproduction* 14 (November 1999): 2868–71.

Clifford, K., R. Rai, and L. Regan. "Future pregnancy outcome in unexplained recurrent first-trimester miscarriage." *Human Reproduction* 12 (1997): 387–89.

U.S. Centers for Disease Control and Prevention. "Known health effects for DES daughters." *DES Update: Consumers.* http://www.cdc.gov/des/consumers/about/effects_daughters.html.

Testing

Tal, J., et al. "A possible role for activated protein C resistance in patients with first- and second-trimester pregnancy failure." *Human Reproduction* 14 (June 1999): 1624–27.

Treatment

HEPARIN

Di Nisio, M., L. W. Peters, and S. Middeldorp. "Anticoagulants for the treatment of recurrent pregnancy loss in women without antiphospholipid syndrome." *Cochrane Database of Systematic Reviews* 3 (2006).

Girardi, G., P. Redecha, and J. E. Salmon. "Heparin prevents antiphospholipid antibody-induced fetal loss by inhibiting complement activation." *Nature Medicine* 10 (October 2004): 1222–26.

Hills, F. A., et al. "Heparin prevents programmed cell death in human trophoblast." *Molecular Human Reproduction* 12 (March 2006): 237–43.

U.S. National Library of Medicine and National Institutes of Health. "Heparin Injection." *MedlinePlus.* http://www.nlm.nih.gov/medlineplus/druginfo/medmaster/a682826.html.

LOW-DOSE ASPIRIN

Rai, R., et al. "Randomised controlled trial of aspirin and aspirin plus heparin in pregnant women with recurrent miscarriage associated with phospholipid antibodies (or antiphospholipid antibodies)." *British Medical Journal* 314 (1997): 253.

Rai, R., et al. "Recurrent miscarriage—an aspirin a day?" *Human Reproduction* 15 (October 2000): 2220–23.

PROGESTERONE SUPPLEMENTS

Arck, P. "Stress and embryo implantation." *Journal of Gynecology, Obstretrics, and Biological Reproduction* 33 (February 2004): 40–42.

Arck, P. C. "Stress and pregnancy loss: role of immune mediators, hormones, and neurotransmitters." *American Journal of Reproductive Immunology* 46 (August 2001): 117–23.

Daya, S. "Efficacy of progesterone support for pregnancy in women with recurrent miscarriage. A meta-analysis of controlled trials." *British Journal of Gynaecology* 96 (March 1989): 275.

Oates-Whitehead, R. M., D. M. Haas, and J. A. K. Carrier. "Progestogen for preventing miscarriage." *Cochrane Database of Systematic Reviews* 2 (2005).

Clomid (Clomiphene Citrate)

Dickey, R. P., S. N. Taylor, D. N . Curole, P. H. Rye, and R. Pyrzak. "Infertility: Incidence of spontaneous abortion in clomiphene pregnancies." *Human Reproduction* 11 (1996): 2623–28.

Ginsberg, K. A. "Luteal-phase defect: etiology, diagnosis, and management." *Endocrinology and Metabolism Clinics of North America* 21 (March 1992): 85–104.

Folic Acid and B Vitamins

Antony, A. C. "Vegetarianism and vitamin B_{12} (cobalamin) deficiency." *American Journal of Clinical Nutrition* 78 (2003): 3–6.

Bennett, M. "Vitamin B_{12} deficiency, infertility, and recurrent fetal loss." *Journal of Reproductive Medicine* 46 (March 2001): 209–12.

De la Calle, M., et al. "Homocysteine, folic acid, and B-group vitamins in obstetrics and gynaecology." *European Journal of Obstetrics, Gynecology, and Reproductive Biology* 107 (April 2003): 125–34.

George, L., et al. "Plasma folate levels and risk of spontaneous abortion." *Journal of the American Medical Association* 288 (October 2002): 1867–73.

Lumley, J., L. Watson, M. Watson, and C. Bower. "Periconceptional supplementation with folate and/or multivitamins for preventing neural tube defects." *Cochrane Library* 2 (2006).

Reznikoff-Etievant, M .F., et al. "Low vitamin B_{12} level as a risk factor for very early recurrent abortion." *European Journal of Obstetrics, Gynecology, and Reproductive Biology* 104 (September 2002): 156–59.

Van der Put, et al. "Folate, homocysteine and neural tube defects: an overview." *Experimental Biology and Medicine* 226 (2001): 243–70.

Prednisone

Hooper, R. "Is steroid treatment for miscarriage safe?" *New Scientist* 186 (June 2005): 17.

Østensen, M. E., and J. F. Skomsvoll. "Anti-inflammatory pharmacotherapy during pregnancy." *Expert Opinion on Pharmacotherapy* 5 (March 2004): 571–80.

U.S. National Library of Medicine and National Institutes of Health. "Prednisone." *MedlinePlus.* http://www.nlm.nih.gov/medlineplus/druginfo/medmaster/a601102.html.

Metformin

Brown, F. M., et al. "Metformin in pregnancy." *Diabetes Care* 29 (2006): 485–86.

Glueck, C. J., et al. "Height, weight, and motor-social development during the first 18 months of life in 126 infants born to 109 mothers with polycystic ovary syndrome who conceived on and continued metformin through pregnancy." *Human Reproduction* 19 (June 2004): 1323–30.

Glueck, C. J., et al. "Pregnancy outcomes among women with polycystic ovary syndrome treated with metformin." *Human Reproduction* 17 (November 2002): 2858–64.

Jakubowicz, D. J., et al. "Effects of metformin on early pregnancy loss in the polycystic ovary syndrome." *Journal of Clinical Endocrinology & Metabolism* 87 (2002): 524–29.

U.S. National Libraries of Medicine and National Institutes of Health. "Metformin." *MedlinePlus.* http://www.nlm.nih.gov/medlineplus/druginfo/medmaster/a696005.html.

Intravenous Immunoglobulin (IVIg)

Carp, H. J. A., et al. "Further experience with intravenous immunoglobulin in women with recurrent miscarriage and a poor prognosis." *American Journal of Reproductive Immunology* 46 (October 2001): 268–73.

Christiansen, O. B., et al. "A randomized, double-blind, placebo-controlled trial of intravenous immunoglobulin in the prevention of recurrent miscarriage: evidence for a therapeutic effect in women with secondary recurrent miscarriage." *Human Reproduction* 17 (March 2002): 809–16.

Jablonowska, B., et al. "Prevention of recurrent spontaneous abortion by intravenous immunoglobulin: a double-blind placebo-controlled study." *Human Reproduction* 14 (March 1999): 838–41.

Porter, T. F., Y. LaCoursiere, and J. R. Scott. "Immunotherapy for recurrent miscarriage." *Cochrane Database of Systematic Reviews* 3 (2006).

Sher, G., et al. "The selective use of heparin/aspirin therapy, alone or in combination with intravenous immunoglobulin in the management of antiphospholipid antibody positive women undergoing in vitro fertilization." *American Journal of Reproductive Immunology* 40 (1998): 74–82.

Stricker, R. B., A. Steinleitner, and E. E. Winger. "Intravenous immunoglobulin (IVIg) therapy for immunologic abortion." *Clinical and Applied Immunology* Reviews 2 (2002): 187–99.

Paternal Leukocyte Immunization

Christiansen, O. B., H. S. Nielsen, and B. Pedersen. "Active or passive immunization in unexplained recurrent miscarriage." *Journal of Reproductive Immunology* 62 (June 2004): 41–52.

Clark, D. A., et al. "Unexplained sporadic and recurrent miscarriage in the new millennium: a critical analysis of immune mechanisms and treatments." *Human Reproduction Update* 7 (2001): 501–11.

Pandey, M. K., S. Thakur, and S. Agrawai. "Lymphocyte immunotherapy and its probable mechanism in the maintenance of pregnancy in women with recurrent spontaneous abortion." *Archives of Gynecology and Obstetrics* 269 (March 2004): 161–72.

Porter, T. F., Y. LaCoursiere, and J. R. Scott. "Immunotherapy for recurrent miscarriage." *Cochrane Database of Systematic Reviews* 3 (2006).

Bromocriptine

Hirahara, F., et al. "Hyperprolactinemic recurrent miscarriage and results of randomized bromocriptine treatment trials." *Fertility & Sterility* 70 (August 1998): 246–52.

Human Chorionic Gonadotropin Injections

Harrison, R. F. "Treatment of habitual abortion with human chorionic gonadotropin: results of open and placebo-controlled studies." *European Journal of Obstetrics, Gynecology, and Reproductive Biology* 20 (September 1985): 159–68.

Pearce, J. M. and R. I. Hamid. "Randomised controlled trial of the use of human chorionic gonadotrophin in recurrent miscarriage associated with polycystic ovaries." *British Journal of Obstetrics and Gynaecology* 101 (August 1994): 685–88.

Quenby, S., and R. G. Farquharson. "Human chorionic gonadotropin supplementation in recurring pregnancy loss: a controlled trial." *Fertility & Sterility* 62 (1994): 708–10.

Preimplantation Genetic Diagnosis

Vidal, F., et al. "Is there a place for preimplantation genetic diagnosis screening in recurrent miscarriage patients?" *Journal of Reproduction and Fertility Supplement* 55 (2000): 143–46.

Wilton, L. "Preimplantation genetic diagnosis for aneuploidy screening in early human embryos: a review." *Prenatal Diagnosis* 22 (June 2002): 512–18.

Cerclage

Ayers, J. W., E. P. Peterson, and R. Ansbacher. "Early therapy for the incompetent cervix in patients with habitual abortion." *Fertility & Sterility* 38 (August 1982): 177–81.

Bachmann, L. M., et al. "Elective cervical cerclage for prevention of preterm birth: a systematic review." *Acta Obstetricia et Gynecologica Scandinavica* 82 (May 2003): 398–404.

Drakeley, A. J., D. Roberts, and Z. Alfirevic. "Cervical cerclage for prevention of preterm delivery: meta-analysis of randomized trials." *Obstetrics & Gynecology* 102 (2003): 621–27.

MacDougall, J., and N. Siddle. "Emergency cervical cerclage." *British Journal of Obstetrics & Gynecology* 98 (December 1991): 1234.

Supportive Care

Clifford, K., R. Rai, and L. Regan. "Future pregnancy outcome in unexplained recurrent first trimester miscarriage." *Human Reproduction* 12 (1997): 387–89.

Lidell, H. S., N. S. Pattison, and A. Zanderigo. "Recurrent miscarriage—outcome after supportive care in early pregnancy." *Australia and New Zealand Journal of Obstetrics and Gynaecology* 31 (November 1991): 320–22.

Surrogacy

Raziel, A., et al. "Successful pregnancy after 24 consecutive fetal losses: lessons learned from surrogacy." *Fertility & Sterility* 74 (July 2000): 104–6.

Van den Akker, O. "Genetic and gestational surrogate mothers' experience of surrogacy." *Journal of Reproductive and Infant Psychology* 21 (May 2003): 145–61.

CHAPTER 4

Dietary Changes

Chrysohoou, C., et al. "Adherence to the Mediterranean diet attenuates inflammation and coagulation process in healthy adults." *Journal of the American College of Cardiology* 44 (2004): 152–58.

Hu, F. B., et al. "Diet, lifestyle, and the risk of type 2 diabetes mellitus in women." *New England Journal of Medicine* 345 (September 2001): 790–97.

Michels, K. B., and A. Wolk. "A prospective study of variety of healthy foods and mortality in women." *International Journal of Epidemiology* 31 (2002): 847–54.

Ryan, M., et al. "Diabetes and the Mediterranean diet: a beneficial effect of oleic acid on insulin sensitivity, adipocyte glucose transport and endothelium-dependent vasoreactivity." *Quarterly Journal of Medicine* 93 (2000): 85–91.

Weidner, G., et al. "Improvements in hostility and depression in relation to dietary change and cholesterol lowering. The family heart study." *Annals of Internal Medicine* 117 (November 1992): 820–23.

Nutritional Supplements

Güvenç, M., et al. "Low levels of selenium in miscarriage." *Journal of Trace Elements in Experimental Medicine* 15 (April 2002): 97–101.

Henmi, H., et al. "Effects of ascorbic acid supplementation on serum progesterone levels in patients with a luteal-phase defect." *Fertility and Sterility* 80 (August 2003): 459–61.

Kumar, K. S. D., et al. "Role of red cell selenium in recurrent pregnancy loss." *Journal of Obstetrics and Gynecology* 22 (March 2002): 181–83.

Rosa, F. W., A. L. Wilk, and F. O. Kelsey. "Vitamin A congeners." *Teratology* 33 (May 2005): 355–64.

Rumbold, A., P. Middleton, and C. A. Crowther. "Vitamin supplementation for preventing miscarriage." *Cochrane Database of Systematic Reviews* 3 (2006).

Acupuncture

Li, J., and X. Gan-gong. "Development of acupuncture treatment and clinical research of threatened abortion." *World Journal of Acupuncture-Moxibustion* 15 (2000): 54–57.

Mayer, D. J. "Acupuncture: an evidence-based review of the clinical literature." *Annual Review of Medicine* 51 (February 2000): 49–63.

National Center for Complementary and Alternative Medicine. "Acupuncture." *Health Information: Treatment or Therapy.* http://nccam.nih.gov/health/acupuncture/.

Paulus, W. E., et al. "Influence of acupuncture on the pregnancy rate in patients who undergo assisted reproduction therapy." *Fertility and Sterility* 77 (April 2002): 721–24.

White, A., et al. "Adverse events following acupuncture: prospective survey of 32,000 consultations with doctors and physiotherapists." *British Medical Journal* 323 (September 2001): 485–86.

Herbal Medicine

Hussin, A. H. "Adverse effects of herbs and drug-herbal interactions." *Malaysian Journal of Pharmacy* 1 (2001): 39–44.

Herbs2000.com. "False unicorn." http://www.herbs2000.com/herbs/herbs_false_unicorn.htm.

Weight Loss

Clark, A. M., et al. "Weight loss in obese infertile women results in improvement in reproductive outcome for all forms of fertility treatment." *Human Reproduction* 13 (1998): 1502–5.

Yoga and Meditation

Astin, J. A. "Stress reduction through mindfulness meditation. Effects on psychological symptomatology, sense of control, and spiritual experiences." *Psychotherapy and Psychosomatics* 66 (1997): 97–106.

Berger, B. G., and D. R. Owen. "Mood alteration with yoga and swimming: aerobic exercise may not be necessary." *Perceptual and Motor Skills* 75 (December 1992): 1331–43.

Davidson, R. J., et al. "Alterations in brain and immune function produced by mindfulness meditation." *Psychosomatic Medicine* 65 (2003): 564–70.

Machanda, S. C., et al. "Retardation of coronary atherosclerosis with yoga lifestyle intervention." *Journal of the Association of Physicians of India* 48 (July 2000): 687–94.

MacLean, C. R., et al. "Effects of the transcendental meditation program on adaptive mechanisms: changes in hormone levels and responses to stress after 4 months of practice." *Psychoneuroendocrinology* 22 (May 1997): 277–95.

Sudsuang, R., V. Chentanez, and K. Veluvan. "Effect of Buddhist meditation on serum cortisol and total protein levels, blood pressure, pulse rate, lung volume, and reaction time." *Physiology & Behavior* 50 (1991): 435–48.

Sundar, S., et al. "Role of yoga in management of essential hypertension." *Acta Cardiology* 39 (1984): 203–8.

Homeopathy

Endrizzi, C., et al. "Harm in homeopathy: aggravations, adverse drug events or medication errors?" *Homeopathy* 94 (October 2005): 233–40.

Kirby, B. J. "Safety of homeopathic products." *Journal of the Royal Society of Medicine* 95 (May 2002): 221–22.

CHAPTER 5

The Aftermath

Klock, S. C., et al. "Psychological distress among women with recurrent spontaneous abortion." *Psychosomatics* 38 (1997): 503–7.

Prettyman, R. J., C. J. Cordle, and G. D. Cook. "A three-month follow-up of psychological morbidity after early miscarriage." *British Journal of Medical Psychology* 66 (December 1993): 363–72.

Your Relationship with Your Partner

Beutel, M., et al. "Similarities and differences in couples' grief reactions following a miscarriage: results from a longitudinal study." *Journal of Psychosomatic Research* 40 (March 1996): 245–53.

Cuisinier, M., et al. "Pregnancy following miscarriage; course of grief and some determining factors." *Journal of Psychosomatic Obstetrics and Gynaecology* 17 (September 1996): 168–74.

Swanson, K. M., et al. "Miscarriage effects on couples' interpersonal and sexual relationships during the first year after loss: women's perceptions." *Psychosomatic Medicine* 65 (2003): 902–10.

CHAPTER 6

When Can I Try Again?

Goldstein, R. R., M. S. Croughan, and P. Robertson. "Neonatal outcomes in immediate versus delayed conceptions after spontaneous abortion: A retrospective case series." *American Journal of Obstetrics & Gynecology* 186 (June 2002): 1230–36.

Choosing a Good Prenatal Vitamin-and-Mineral Supplement

Hoag, S. W., H. Ramachandruni, and R. F. Shangraw. "Failure of prescription prenatal vitamin products to meet USP standards for folic acid dissolution." *Journal of the American Pharmacists Association* 37 (1997): 397–400.

March of Dimes. "Before you're pregnant: choosing a multivitamin." http://www.marchofdimes.com/pnhec/173_15354.asp.

Saliva Ovulation Predictor Tests

Berardono, B., et al. "Is the salivary 'ferning' a reliable index of the fertile period?" *Acta European Fertility* 24 (1993): 61–65.

CHAPTER 7

Seeing the Heartbeat

Brigham, S. A., C. Conlon, and R. G. Farquharson. "A longitudinal study of pregnancy outcome following idiopathic recurrent miscarriage." *Human Reproduction* 14 (November 1999): 2868–71.

Hill, L. M., et al. "Fetal loss rate after ultrasonically documented cardiac activity between 6 and 14 weeks, menstrual age." *Journal of Clinical Ultrasound* 19 (May 1991): 221–23.

Hyer, J. S., et al. "Predictive value of the presence of an embryonic heartbeat for live birth: comparison of women with and without recurrent pregnancy loss." *Fertility and Sterility* 82 (November 2004): 1369–73.

Van Lith, J. M. M., et al. "Fetal heart rate in early pregnancy and chromosomal disorders." *British Journal of Obstetrics & Gynecology* 99 (September 1992): 741.

If You Have Vaginal Bleeding or Spotting

Strobino, B., and J. Pantel-Silverman. "Gestational vaginal bleeding and pregnancy outcome." *American Journal of Epidemiology* 129 (1989): 806–15.

Ultrasound

Nordqvist, C. "Ultrasound might affect newborn brain development." *MedicalNewsToday.*
http://www.medicalnewstoday.com/healthnews.php?newsid=49122.

Nuchal Translucency Test and Ultra-Screen

NTD Laboratories, Inc. "Ultra-Screen (first trimester)."
http://www.ntdlabs.com/patient_usf.php.

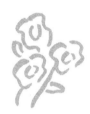

Index